Nursing Knowledge and Theory Innovation

Pamela G. Reed, PhD, RN, FAAN, is a professor at the University of Arizona College of Nursing. Her research, practice, and scholarship focus on well-being and mental health across the life span, nursing metatheory and philosophy, and ethics and spirituality in end-of-life nursing care. Dr. Reed's self-transcendence theory is published in several nursing theory textbooks and articles, and has been used widely in research and practice. In addition, her Spiritual Perspective Scale and Self-Transcendence Scale have been used by researchers around the world. Dr. Reed teaches philosophy, metatheory, and middle range nursing theory development to doctoral nursing students in DNP and PhD academic programs, and she has received numerous awards for outstanding teaching. In addition to her many publications, she, along with coauthor Nelma Shearer, has published three editions of *Perspectives in Nursing Theory*. Dr. Reed is a fellow in the American Academy of Nursing.

Nelma B. Crawford Shearer, PhD, RN, FAAN, is an associate professor emeritus and former director of the Hartford Center of Gerontological Nursing Excellence at Arizona State University College of Nursing and Health Innovation. She is a fellow in the American Academy of Nursing. During her career, Dr. Shearer focused extensively on developing, testing, and disseminating a community-based intervention for older adults derived from her theory of health empowerment. Her work has been published in both research and clinical practice journals as part of her ongoing commitment to clinical practice issues and the development of clinically relevant theory for practice. Dr. Shearer's theory-based health empowerment intervention has been cited in publications both nationally and internationally. Dr. Shearer has also received numerous awards for her outstanding scholarship, teaching, and research.

Nursing Knowledge and Theory Innovation

Advancing the Science of Practice

Second Edition

Pamela G. Reed, PhD, RN, FAAN

Nelma B. Crawford Shearer, PhD, RN, FAAN

Editors

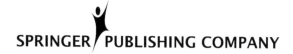
SPRINGER PUBLISHING COMPANY

KH

Springer Publishing Company, LLC
11 West 42nd Street
New York, NY 10036
www.springerpub.com

Acquisitions Editor: Margaret Zuccarini
Compositor: Westchester Publishing Services

ISBN: 978-0-8261-4991-6
ebook ISBN: 978-0-8261-4992-3
Instructor's PowerPoints ISBN: 978-0-8261-4996-1

Instructor's Materials: Qualified instructors may request supplements by emailing textbook@springerpub.com.

17 18 19 20 / 5 4 3 2 1

The author and the publisher of this Work have made every effort to use sources believed to be reliable to provide information that is accurate and compatible with the standards generally accepted at the time of publication. Because medical science is continually advancing, our knowledge base continues to expand. Therefore, as new information becomes available, changes in procedures become necessary. We recommend that the reader always consult current research and specific institutional policies before performing any clinical procedure. The author and publisher shall not be liable for any special, consequential, or exemplary damages resulting, in whole or in part, from the readers' use of, or reliance on, the information contained in this book. The publisher has no responsibility for the persistence or accuracy of URLs for external or third-party Internet websites referred to in this publication and does not guarantee that any content on such websites is, or will remain, accurate or appropriate.

Library of Congress Cataloging-in-Publication Data

Names: Reed, Pamela G., author. | Shearer, Nelma B. Crawford, 1950– author.
Title: Nursing knowledge and theory innovation : advancing the science of practice / Pamela G. Reed, Nelma B. Crawford Shearer.
Description: Second edition. | New York, NY : Springer Publishing Company, LLC, [2018] | Includes bibliographical references and index.
Identifiers: LCCN 2017029181 (print) | LCCN 2017029569 (ebook) | ISBN 9780826149923 (ebook) | ISBN 9780826149916 (hardcopy : alk. paper) | ISBN 9780826149961 (Instructors PowerPoints)
Subjects: | MESH: Nursing Theory | Nurse's Role | Practice Patterns, Nurses' | Health Knowledge, Attitudes, Practice
Classification: LCC RT81.5 (ebook) | LCC RT81.5 (print) | NLM WY 86 | DDC 610.73—dc23
LC record available at https://lccn.loc.gov/2017029181

Printed in the United States of America by McNaughton & Gunn.

4/9/18

We dedicate this book to our students and colleagues who share our interest in the synergy within the science and practice of nursing.

Contents

Contributors

Barbara B. Brewer, PhD, RN, MALS, MBA, FAAN, Associate Professor, The University of Arizona, College of Nursing, Tucson, Arizona

Catherine Johnson, PhD, PNP, FNP, Assistant Professor, Duquesne University, School of Nursing, Pittsburgh, Pennsylvania

Rene Love, PhD, DNP, PMHNP-BC, FNAP, FAANP, Clinical Associate Professor, Director of DNP Program, The University of Arizona, College of Nursing, Tucson, Arizona

Donna Behler McArthur, PhD, APRN, FNP-BC, FAANP, FNAP, Clinical Professor, Director, The University of Arizona, College of Nursing, Tucson, Arizona

Cathleen Michaels, PhD, RN, FNAP, FAAN, Clinical Associate Professor, The University of Arizona, College of Nursing, Tucson, Arizona

Pamela G. Reed, PhD, MSN, MA, RN, FAAN, Professor, The University of Arizona, College of Nursing, Tucson, Arizona

Gary Rolfe, PhD, MA, BSc, RMN, PGCEA, Professor of Nursing, School of Health Science, Swansea University, Swansea, Wales

Jennifer Ruel, DNP, RN, FNP-BC, ENP-BC, Associate Clinical Professor, University of Detroit Mercy, School of Nursing, Detroit, Michigan

Nelma B. Crawford Shearer, PhD, RN, FAAN, Associate Professor Emeritus, Arizona State University, College of Nursing and Health Innovation, Phoenix, Arizona

Donna M. Velasquez, PhD, RN, FNP-BC, FAANP, Clinical Associate Professor, Director, Doctor of Nursing Practice Program, Arizona State University, College of Nursing and Health Innovation, Phoenix, Arizona

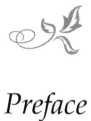

Preface

How is nursing knowledge generated? This is not a new question nor can it be answered simply by referring to the scientific method or evidence-based practice. The increasing number of doctoral-level practicing nurses compels us to revisit this question from new perspectives, particularly the science of nursing practice. Philosophy, science, theory, and practice exist in a complex relationship that generates knowledge in and for nursing. The burgeoning of doctoral-level practicing nurses presents new opportunities for building nursing knowledge to meet society's health care needs.

This book is unique in its contribution to the theory textbook literature with its goal of expanding nursing's knowledge-generating capacity by engaging nurses in theory and knowledge development through their practice lenses—from the practice experiences and expertise they bring to their scholarly work. Scholars within and outside of nursing are calling for the practice dimension of the discipline to play a more active role in developing new knowledge.

The 15 chapters in this book present philosophical, historical, practical, and theoretical perspectives regarding practice-centered knowledge development. Theory innovation, in terms of the development and creative application of conceptual dimensions of knowledge, is a thread throughout the book. Five chapters were developed as *Interludes* where readers can pause and explore specific aspects of knowledge development in reference to their own nursing practice and research. An important feature of the book is its philosophical stance on the practice turn in theory and knowledge development, and the encouragement and guidance for nurses to regard practice as a context for both the development and application of nursing theory.

This second edition features important updates across all chapters, along with a reorganization of the original first chapter into two chapters to better describe the roles of theory and the philosophical "Isms" as relevant perspectives in knowledge development. *Intermodernism* is featured as a philosophy of nursing science and practice that synthesizes important tenets of other philosophical views. The book also introduces two new chapters, each of which pushes current thinking forward in expanding our capacity to develop knowledge. "The DNP Project: Translating Research Into Knowledge for Practice" (Chapter 6) promotes development of practice knowledge through a dual process of scholarship in the practice of nursing and the practice of science. The chapter discusses knowledge translation in terms relevant to the doctor of nursing practice (DNP) project, and presents models along with specific guidelines for the DNP project process. The goal of the chapter "Generating Knowledge in Practice: Philosophical and Methodological Considerations" (Chapter 11) is to guide and encourage nurses to be knowledge generators by engaging in practice-based evidence research in settings where they may practice or teach, from point-of-care with patients to system-level health care. It also addresses ethical and epistemic considerations as rationales for the move to practice-based evidence research beyond traditional evidence-based practice procedures. Summary Points have been added at the end of each chapter, in addition to Questions for Reflection that help reinforce knowledge.

This textbook is intended for graduate-level nursing students, particularly students enrolled in DNP and PhD programs who bring practice into their research and scholarship. It will also be useful for nurse practitioner students or master's-level nursing students enrolled in a theory course or planning their master's research projects. Doctorally prepared nurses and faculty will also find this book relevant in their scholarly work.

In sharing the ideas in this book, we seek to inspire and equip nursing students with the tools to make theory more relevant to their own practice, to become aware of and develop their own theoretical ideas in practice, and, in doing so, advance practice while building confidence in their own knowledge. Recognition of the theoretical thinking that occurs within evidence-based practice invites continued dialogue concerning how we think about nurses' scholarly practice and how we educate nurses at graduate and doctoral levels.

Pamela G. Reed
Nelma B. Crawford Shearer

Acknowledgments

Many people have contributed to making this book a success for nursing. We first want to acknowledge our eight contributors, whose expertise and creative scholarship in nursing are recorded between the covers of this book. Their chapters provide unique insights through the practice lens for exploring new thinking about knowledge development in nursing.

We also sincerely appreciate everyone at Springer Publishing Company for their careful, expert work in transforming ideas about theory innovation and knowledge development in nursing practice and science into this portable package. We especially thank Margaret Zuccarini, acquisitions editor at Springer Publishing Company, for championing both editions of our book to the editorial board, and for her wisdom and encouragement throughout the project. We also acknowledge Amanda Devine, assistant editor at Springer Publishing Company, for her patient guidance and abiding attention to detail in pulling everything together.

Last, we express deep gratitude to our students, past and present, at the University of Arizona and Arizona State University who helped inspire the creation of this book. It is our hope that the chapters will further students' learning and equip them with the tools to make theory more relevant to their own practice, to develop their own theoretical ideas in practice, and, in so doing, advance practice while building nursing knowledge.

1

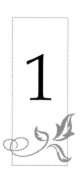

The Spiral Path of Nursing Knowledge

Pamela G. Reed

Theory texts present creative and scholarly applications of theory to practice. This focus on *application*, not *origination*, of theory in practice has occurred partly out of our scientific heritage where knowledge is traditionally regarded as a rational, cognitive process separate from the social and practical (and messy!) contexts in which it is used (e.g., Longino, 2002, 2008). So, theories have come into our practice and research more or less ready-made, having been developed in a so-called rational, cognitive context of, say, an armchair. However, shifts in philosophy of science—generally and in nursing specifically—are bringing together in more deliberate ways the development, translation, and application of knowledge, which paves the way for theory innovation. Further, Stehr (2004) has reminded us that the *amount* of knowledge developed amid the proliferation of research findings and other evidence for practice should be balanced with attention to *how* knowledge is developed. Thus, a frontier in knowledge development is the production of knowledge and theory in the patient-centered context of nursing practice.

It is generally thought that researchers and theorists provide new knowledge and theories for practicing nurses to apply, evaluate, and perhaps modify in their practice. Granted, nurses do look within their practice, for example, in terms of their keen observations, interactions with patients and families, conversations with colleagues, and expert judgment to inform their practice. But nurses have the capacity for theoretical thinking as well as research to develop scientific knowledge *for* practice *in* practice. The science of practice holds the potential for interested nurses to generate knowledge through scientific inquiry, practice-based interactions, and innovative theoretical thinking.

A CALL FOR TRANSFORMATION

The ideas expressed across the chapters in this book converge with four key recommendations for educating nurses outlined by Benner, Sutphen, Leonard, and Day (2010) in their call for radical transformation of nursing programs. That is, this book encourages development of contextualized knowledge for practice; promotes more deliberate strategies to link theory to practice; supports the emphasis on clinical scholarship in exploring new ways of reasoning and theorizing in practice beyond the focus on critical thinking; and supports the transformation of practicing nurses' identity by encouraging and guiding their participation as knowledge producers beyond that of knowledge users in practice. Further, innovative theoretical thinking in practice and the various knowledge sources from which it draws must not be eclipsed by any of the more familiar reasoning processes of critical thinking, evidence-based practice (EBP) procedures, problem solving, or decision making (Lester & Piore, 2004).

THEORETICAL HERITAGE IN NURSING

In the late 19th century, Britain's Florence Nightingale professionalized nursing practice by enacting her theoretical ideas about the significance of the physical and social environments in human health and well-being. Nightingale's focus on facilitating the person's inner processes of healing by tending to the environment, along with her expertise in statistics and other ways of knowing, made her a compelling leader for nursing science and practice. As the 20th century progressed, new leaders in theoretical thinking energized nursing's advancement in education, research, and practice. Hildegard Peplau's (1952) theory of interpersonal relations introduced a major scientific treatise on the nurse–patient relationship, which remains a defining focus of nursing practice. Martha Rogers's (1970) work on the theoretical basis of nursing presented progressive ideas about human complexity and person–environment processes that are still unfolding today in contemporary theorizing and science. Many other notable theorists—including some of you—have joined and will join these three historical icons to advance the role of nursing in the knowledge and practice of health care.

Nursing has a rich history of theoretical thinkers. Nursing scientist scholars who were first educated in theory-based or theory-enriched disciplines like sociology, psychology, anthropology, and education provided an abundance of theoretical thinking and conceptual systems of, and for, nursing. Nurses educated in graduate-level nursing programs followed and produced theories and theory-related writings about nursing. Because of this, we may take for granted what some fields (e.g., McQueen, 2007) still quest for—a theoretical basis for the profession.

The purpose of this chapter is to present a Path of Nursing Knowledge to encourage and guide participation among nurses, particularly practicing nurses, in developing knowledge for the discipline. It is a path *of*, rather than *to*, knowledge because there is no ultimate goal or final theory in knowledge development. The theories of today need to be sensitive to the given situation and changing problems and experiences, yet also illuminate patterns that broaden understanding of nursing phenomena. The Path offers up a tentative yet useful form of knowledge called "theories," but invariably spirals us forward through the process of knowledge building.

The linchpin of this path is the *practice of nursing*, that is, facilitating *processes of health and well-being within and among human systems across a diversity of environments* (Reed, 1997). The integral link between practice and knowledge is not new, and emphasizing this link in nursing's network of knowledge presents some challenges for science and theory innovation. However, the challenges are worthwhile given their potential for furthering nursing's unique and innovative contributions to human health and health care. This and the next chapter are a beginning in what I hope will become an extended dialogue about innovations in developing nursing knowledge. Authors of subsequent chapters take up the dialogue from their various practices and perspectives.

THE SPIRAL PATH

Along the hiking trails in mountains where the ancients once walked, you can spot petroglyphs, ancient carvings or inscriptions, embedded in the rocks and boulders. Some of these depict a spiral form, which is found on every continent. I used this spiral form to symbolize a process of knowledge development in nursing (see Figure 1.1). To the ancient people, the spiral form represented one of various ideas that can apply to the process of knowledge development: an energy; a life-giving source like water; a process of emerging or transcending; a portal or gateway from the mundane to the eternal realms; or perhaps most relevant to the career of being a nursing student or scholar is its symbolization of a life journey and the challenges for growth faced along the way.

The petroglyph that inspired the spiral design resembles a foot path, earthy and imperfect, of various turns. It is not a perfect spiral like the artificial depiction you might find in a catalog, but rather, it is imperfect to represent the natural, dynamic, and often messy processes of nursing practice, science, and theorizing.

The spiral path has six turns over the geography of nursing knowledge. Each turn corresponds to a particular focus and tool of inquiry for knowledge development. The components of the Path are not arranged hierarchically, unlike other models of the structure of nursing knowledge. Instead, the spiral is an ongoing and nonlinear path, open to influences that can be incorporated for innovative and unpredictable change. The Path, rather than being a series of concentric circles, is a spiral form to convey continuity across the dimensions; from everyday knowledge work to scientific theories, knowledge construction is a "fundamentally continuous" process, as described by the practicing scientist Fleck in his book on comparative epistemology, *Genesis and Development of a Science Fact* (cited in Smith, 2005, p. 26).

The spiral path is a way of thinking about how various components of knowledge development are organized and related. What are listed here may be modified or expanded, depending on your context of nursing science and practice, and depending on what you would like to emphasize—a pragmatic turn? an ethical turn? or a spiritual turn? It is likely, though, that any approach to knowledge development involves a dynamic network or web of components that includes philosophical, empirical, and theoretical dimensions of the discipline.

Knowledge development is, above all, an emergent process, paralleling the process of change that its creators undergo over time—open and ongoing, developmental and sometimes decremental, patterned yet unpredictable, complex yet organized, bringing forth outcomes that are greater than the sum of its various turns, but still influenced by each turn. The scientific knowledge produced, as indicated by the *theory* circle, is not necessarily cumulative nor is it unchanging or unchangeable, but it is relevant to the practice situation or problems to which it is linked. And of course, other forms of knowledge inhabit the path. Nursing knowledge is enriched by many patterns of knowing, which inform, and are informed by, the scientific pattern represented by the theory component of the Path.

THE CONTEXTS OF THEORY

Theory is a central component in the Path of Nursing Knowledge. Theory is the "vehicle of scientific knowledge, and one way or another become[s] involved in most aspects of the scientific enterprise" (Suppe, 1977, p. 3). Theory exists within a context of philosophical, empirical, and theoretical dimensions, and has a path of inquiry whereby theory emerges out of nursing practice and research. Theory also functions reflexively to inform nurses' practice and research. This path of inquiry is represented in Figure 1.1, which highlights key aspects of the philosophical, empirical, and theoretical dimensions of knowledge development.

Philosophical Dimension

The philosophical dimension consists of conceptual components that influence knowledge development, including philosophy of science, the nursing metaparadigm, and

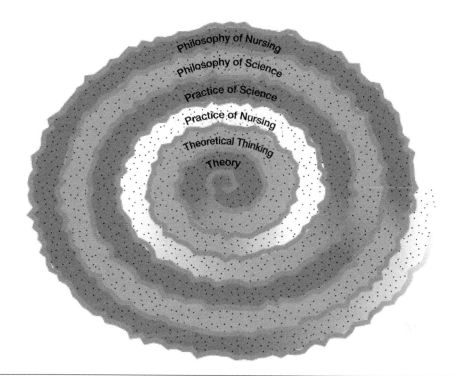

Philosophy of Nursing
Philosophy of Science
Practice of Science
Practice of Nursing
Theoretical Thinking
Theory

FIGURE 1.1 The Spiral Path of Nursing Knowledge.

philosophy of nursing, as well as personal beliefs and values. These philosophical components express the conceptual perspectives that influence (or at least are related to) the *substantive* focus of theories (ontology) and the *process* focus on empirical methods and patterns of knowing and warranting knowledge (epistemology) in a discipline. The philosophical dimension broadly describes the way things are from a certain perspective of reality, and the way things should be from a certain perspective of morality. In Figure 1.1, these dimensions are represented by the *philosophy of nursing* and the *philosophy of science*.

Empirical Dimension

The empirical components are the observables used in knowledge generation as obtained directly or indirectly through the senses, for example, through the nurse's personal life experiences, nursing practice and other professional experiences, the patient's assessed needs and perspectives, research methods of observation and measurement of variables in the theory, and empirical findings from research. Of course, because our body and mind are *not* distinct Cartesian entities, anything obtained through the senses is already interpreted, as influenced by conceptual (philosophical and theoretical) dimensions. These dimensions, represented by the *practice of science* and the *practice of nursing* in Figure 1.1, sit between the philosophical and theoretical dimensions in the Path, as shown in the figure because these material, embodied practices are considered to be a linchpin in nursing knowledge development.

Theoretical Dimension

The theoretical dimension in this Path of Nursing Knowledge involves both a process and product, that is, *theoretical thinking* and the conceptual structure called a *theory*, respectively, as represented toward the center of the Path in Figure 1.1. Theories are open systems, which are amendable to change and possible improvement by critique, modification, and refinement through ongoing theory development and evaluation. Theory development is influenced by both the philosophical and empirical dimensions. Theories link the everyday world of practice and the philosophical perspectives of reality.

METATHEORY

Metatheory is a word that ties together the three areas addressed in the Path. Metatheory refers to the area of study of the philosophical, theoretical, and empirical components and their relationships within the structure of knowledge. It is a term used in many disciplines, and sometimes refers to an overarching theory. But most often it is used, as described here, in the broader philosophical context of knowledge development rather than as a specific theoretical perspective. Metatheory is not a scientific theory per se but rather a domain of conceptual tools that inform development of substantive theory, theoretical concepts, and research design.

Nursing metatheory identifies the domain of nursing that addresses the philosophical perspectives, substantive focuses, and methods concerning nursing knowledge. *Metatheory* encompasses all of the elements that are used in developing nursing knowledge, especially the following: philosophies and methods of science; nursing ontology and epistemology; the nursing metaparadigm and the conceptual models that elaborate on the metaparadigm concepts; middle range and other levels of theories; and the nurses' personal values and professional practice domains (Reed, 2010). These metatheoretical tools inform and influence the development of theories and theoretical concepts (Sibeon, 2007).

It is important to attend to these metatheoretical components, which are represented in the Path of Nursing Knowledge, because they account for the human context of science. While theory and knowledge development are addressed here as primarily scientific activities, nonetheless they are human activities—replete with personal values, fallibility, and biases, and influenced by historical, cultural, and social contexts. This fact, along with the inability to remove the challenges and doubts that it interjects into our quest for knowledge, is regarded amusingly by Smith (2005) as *the* scandal of philosophy of science, and it has nearly paralyzed the creativity and productivity of some philosophers and scientists! But as nurses, we embrace the human messiness of knowledge development, as we do in our nursing interactions with people in the midst of wellness and illness, living and dying. Indeed, the context of discovery is very much a part of the metatheoretical concerns about the development and justification of scientific knowledge and theories. And so, let us take a brief tour around this Path of Nursing Knowledge, one step at a time.

SCIENTIFIC THEORY

Scientific theory resides in the center of the spiral. This position is not an end point but a place that launches the nurse back through the Path to test out and refine theoretical knowledge. Theories consist of concepts and proposed relationships between concepts. They provide explanations of processes proposed to underlie or influence phenomena of interest to a discipline.

Nursing theories are emergent products of a nurse's personal experiences and beliefs, professional activities and practices, philosophy of nursing, and philosophy of science, as well as the skill and strategies nurses use in developing knowledge. Theories are open to critique and change. Writers who disparage theory (e.g., Thomas, 2007) offer worthwhile critique but often criticize from a positivist, and therefore limited, view of theory. Theories provide perspective, specificity to inform action, distinction, and clarity for one's professional identity and also provide a (relatively) secure base from which to connect and collaborate with other disciplines in practice and research.

Theories are practical in that they provide an efficient structure to frame our questions and from which to interpret the findings. Good theories help identify the factors to be studied and the questions to be asked. Theories are like clinical or research instruments; they make evidence "observable" that would otherwise be inaccessible (Weissman, 2008), while at the same time being open to testing and change as more clarity is achieved.

DESCRIBING THEORY

Theories are organizations of nursing concepts and evidence into conceptual structures that help practitioners and researchers see pattern and organization in their activities and make sense of what they observe and discover in their work. Theories by definition have both empirical and abstract dimensions. They consist of concepts and statements of relationships between concepts that point to not only a local process or event but also a possible pattern of which the local event is one example. A theory is a tool for conceptualizing and studying practice problems, proposing explanations and interventions, and testing and refining ideas.

Types of Theories

Theories come in different sizes, so to speak. These range from *conceptual models* and *grand theories* that are broad in scope and focus on a large domain of nursing, to *middle range theories* that address a focused area of research or practice in a discipline, to *situation-specific* and *microlevel theories* that have the narrowest scope and most specific focus (see Higgins & Moore, 2000, for a succinct overview). We should also acknowledge a nascent form of theory Nightingale used so effectively—the *empirical generalization*—discussed in a later chapter. Each type of theory from, for example, the broad conceptual frameworks useful in qualitative research to middle range theories of experimental research, can play an important role in knowledge development.

Middle range theories are the most common theories in science. They have less scope than grand theories or conceptual models, and instead focus on specific health experiences, health and illness problems, or certain patient populations. They are still relatively abstract yet provide some explanations about nursing phenomena. Middle range theories have concepts that can be defined empirically so that the relationships proposed in the theory can be tested or explored empirically, through systematic approaches in practice or other settings. Theories are tested by deriving research questions or hypotheses (propositions) from the theory. Nurses build knowledge by testing theories against observations of the natural world, in practice and elsewhere. *Testing,* from an intermodern perspective (presented in Chapter 2), reflects social and practical values along with some of the epistemic values promoted in modernist science.

Theory as a System

Theories can also be thought of as a system, with a boundary and system conditions, interrelated parts internal to the system, and elements that are external to the system that influence its development (Dubin, 1978). The spiral path has outlined several of these external elements that influence theory, such as the nurse's philosophy and practice. *Modern* perspectives depict the relationship between practice and theory as a linear, one-way course of dissemination of theory to practice. *Intermodernism* (see Chapter 2) depicts a different relationship. It is nonlinear movement where both are changed by the relationship between theory and practice. The relationship is one of transformation rather than dissemination (Latour, 1993). It is important to note that theory and practice are distinct processes because in that way they can generate the change that fosters knowledge development. As a system, then, a theory is dynamic and open to change through research, debate, critique, and its expression in practice.

Theory as Process and Product

THEORY AS A GIFT. As a process, theory is a scholarly way of thinking that stimulates new ideas and illuminates potential connections between ideas. But more than this, theory is a process of interacting with patients in practice, which generates the ideas that are formulated into theories. Theory, then, may be regarded as a gift, given by the situation or encounter with patients in nursing care. The nurse's theorizing, in turn, is a way of appreciating the gifts given by patients, a form of appreciative inquiry.

Nature writer and scholar Kathleen Dean Moore (2010) explained that in living close to the wilderness, she had to learn to accept its gifts—and the way to learn, she said, was to practice. She did this by giving back, through her writing about nature. Nurses, too, live close to wilderness and nature in their daily practice with patients and families. The insights, ideas, and lessons that nurses acquire through their work are gifts. They arise from any place where nursing is practiced—in health-related interactions with patients and their families, colleagues, students, teachers, and friends and family, and in quiet self-reflection. Nurses give back not only through their practice but also by developing the potentialities of the caregiving interactions into theories of new knowledge.

THEORY AS AN ART FORM. As a product, theory can be viewed as an art form. Eisner (1985) said that "all scientific inquiry culminates in the creation of form: taxonomies, theories, frameworks, and concept systems. The scientist, like the artist, must transform the content of his or her imagination into some public, stable form, something that can be shared with others . . ." (p. 26). In this way, theory is viewed as a product that proposes and shares possible explanations or solutions. Nursing theories have a particular form and substantive focus, often providing insights and interpretations on one or more of nursing's metaparadigm concepts. The art of theory involves an abstraction from the concrete experience to inform us about a *pattern* (not just a *part*) of human health.

Theories as Nets

A modern or postpositivist view of theories portrays them as nets tossed out to the sea to catch a part of reality. We cannot catch the entire ocean, so an important first step in theory development is to clarify what part of the ocean is our focus (our ontology), and our methods (epistemology) for designing and deploying our net. The nature of the netting will influence the kind of "truths" that are caught from the ocean. Moreover, an intermodern view of theories regards the nets *as* a relevant social reality. "The net, a web of shifting, intersecting, interacting beliefs and practices, *is* truth" (Ludwik Fleck cited in Smith, 2005, p. 51). Our theories, then, are quite powerful in influencing our experiences and practices with patients.

EVALUATING SCIENTIFIC THEORIES

Evaluating theories is an important process in the Path of knowledge development. Evaluation criteria are useful in judging the merits of a theory and may also be used to guide the development of a theory. As dynamic, humanly constructed structures, theories need to be evaluated by a complex set of criteria that take into account the range of values involved in warranting nursing knowledge. These criteria typically reflect both cognitive (or epistemic) values (which are concerned with justifying the theory as true, rational, accurate) and contextual, practical, moral values (which also warrant the knowledge but in a manner connected more closely to the social dimension of science). Standard epistemic values for theory from modernist science include accuracy, parsimony, consistency, generality, fruitfulness, and objectivity (Kuhn, 1977). From an intermodern perspective of knowledge (see Chapter 2), which is pluralistic in its approach to the values that warrant scientific theory, the list of criteria includes not only traditional normative criteria from philosophy of science, but also criteria from social epistemology—a social, contextual perspective of knowledge production—all of which support the aims of science. The following list, then, combines these sets of criteria for evaluating theories, aligning criteria from traditional philosophy with Longino's (1990, 1995, 2002) *critical contextual empiricist* philosophy of knowledge:

1. *Empirical adequacy:* This is a more liberal criterion than *accuracy,* and refers to agreement between the theory's propositions and the data from research. It should not be used alone, but in context with values represented by other criteria.

2. *Novelty:* This criterion is a modified view of *consistency* or *coherence* such that theories do not necessarily have to be coherent with existing theories and the status quo. Theories that offer new understandings may be desired over accepted theories that perpetuate older views not appropriate or useful in the present context.

3. *Ontological heterogeneity:* This aligns with *parsimony,* but modified to allow for differences regarding what counts as a "real entity," to better represent in a theory the unique and dynamic nature of a human system or situation. Difference is seen as a resource not a failure, and may be preferred over simplicity.

4. *Complexity of interactions/relationships:* This criterion is similar to the modification of *parsimony* (or *simplicity).* But in addition to valuing difference over simplicity, this criterion promotes relatedness, mutual exchange, and interactions among different theoretical ideas such that there is no one single factor or relationship that can explain an entity or process.

5. *Applicability to current human needs:* This criterion aligns (mostly) with *fruitfulness* or *pragmatic adequacy* as we may know it. However, fruitfulness, which typically focuses on a theory's ability to generate new research problems, is modified to focus on a theory's capacity to alleviate human needs and promote health empowerment. Rather than looking inward to science and its inner workings and capacity to generate more hypotheses and ideas, this criterion values looking outward to evaluate the social, technological, and ethical implications (beneficial or harmful) of a theory and its supporting research.

6. *Diffusion of power:* This criterion by Longino is relevant to nursing, given its embeddedness in the health science. This criterion for theory expresses a sociopolitical value for facilitating full participation in knowledge production rather than, for example, having extraordinary requirements for research resources or expertise that may limit access to participation in or use of scientific knowledge.

Overall, then, we do not necessarily want criteria that promote homogeneity and unity in nursing knowledge and theories. There is rarely one causal factor or even one stable set of factors that explains health processes and experiences. Human beings, who comprise nursing's major focus, are complex and dynamic. Where traditional science calls for criteria that tend to eliminate alternative theories in a quest for the one best theory, we instead value a pluralism of theories to explain nursing phenomena and an emancipatory approach that empowers a diversity of nurses to participate in knowledge production through scientific inquiry and production of nursing theories.

PHILOSOPHY OF NURSING

Philosophy of Nursing resides in the outermost circle. The Path one takes can begin anywhere; scholars tell us that all knowledge begins and ends with philosophy. Nurses are philosophers at heart if not in practice. Whenever you wrestle with questions about what is morally right or wrong in a patient care situation, when you reflect on what you believe relative to your choices and actions as a practitioner, teacher, or researcher, when you reflect on what you value and its influence on your science or practice, when you and a patient are faced with gray situations where there is no one right answer or approach—you are engaging in philosophical inquiry whether or not you have been formally prepared in the logic and theory behind it.

Philosophers confront questions that cannot be answered by scientific inquiry, but philosophical inquiry nonetheless can provide a window into understanding what evidence you choose to believe in and why, what health goals you pursue in research, and what health goals and behaviors you value for yourself and your patients.

Reflexivity is an important attitude, from a stance both within and outside the situation, to consider explanations, values, and influences on your beliefs and goals in nursing. You can construct your own philosophy of nursing science by engaging in philosophical inquiry through reflecting on and writing down the following elements: your ontological and epistemological views, your metaparadigmatic statement about nursing, and the personal values and professional and life experiences that may influence these views.

PHILOSOPHICAL INQUIRY

Philosophical inquiry is a tool in knowledge development because it raises awareness of factors that influence or inspire your knowledge development in practice and research. Questioning is a key practice within philosophical inquiry. To question is to "decline to take for granted" (Smith, 2005, p. 7). Some of the purposes of philosophical inquiry are as follows:

- To question seemingly self-evident assumptions, beliefs, values
- To expose hidden assumptions and distorted means of thinking
- To provide a context and comprehensive views of the discipline for research and practice
- To address questions that science cannot address (metaphysical, ontological, epistemological, ethical)
- To help ensure that science does not violate the values of the nursing profession
- To keep the discipline open to change through use of reason and reflection

I can learn something about your philosophy of nursing by asking you to respond to questions like the following: *What is nursing? What are the elements of a human being that nursing should attend to? Which ones are the most important? Is there an underlying order to the universe or is it mostly chaos and we make it seem orderly by the beliefs or research methods we impose on the world? Is there a truth out there or is it found within each individual or group? How do you define health, and is it ethical to apply your definition to patients and research participants? Should values be separated from or included as a part of our scientific methods and criteria?* Philosophers interrogate themselves and others with questions about disciplinary values that have no definitive answer but yet permeate our science and practice. There are questions, for example, that inquire about the morality of promoting compliance, the inherent goodness of health or the nurse–patient relationship, or the scientific value in quantifying suffering, love, or spirituality for scientific study. These questions relate to one of the six areas of philosophical inquiry listed in Box 1.1.

ONTOLOGY

Ontology addresses the substance or subject matter of the discipline, and in so doing, defines entities and processes the discipline regards as real and relevant *focuses* for knowledge development and practice. The term *ontology* has been defined in various ways, but at a nursing disciplinary level it refers broadly to the nature of being (human), environment, human health, and so on. Without an explicit ontology, that is, without a clear picture of what substantive focuses we hold for practice and inquiry, we risk clarity in sense of identity within the discipline and then may end up privileging method and other extraneous factors over substance in our inquiry and knowledge development (Yanchar & Hill, 2003).

BOX 1.1 Areas of Philosophical Inquiry

---

1. *Metaphysics:* nature of reality, existence, and substance of the universe
   What is the nature of existence, reality, time, space, causality, and so on, beyond the empirical?

2. *Ontology:* nature of being of a discipline
   What is the focus or substance of a discipline?

3. *Epistemology:* nature of knowledge and truth
   How is knowledge formed and warranted in a given discipline?

4. *Axiology:* nature of values in science
   How does the science handle values in its practice and science?

5. *Ethics:* nature of goodness and human conduct
   What ethical theories and moral views influence disciplinary practices?

6. *Aesthetics:* nature of beauty
   What is considered "beauty" in nursing? Is being healthy beauty? Are the practices of nursing expressions of art?

Metaparadigm

The broadest ontological element is the *metaparadigm*. The metaparadigm is a highly abstract framework that outlines the central focuses of knowledge development in a discipline. The nursing metaparadigm—at least currently—consists of four concepts: person, health, environment, and nursing practice. It is open to change!

The nursing metaparadigm originated in the early 1970s with nurses in education and curriculum development. Lorraine Walker (1971) defined nursing in terms of (a) the persons providing care, (b) persons receiving care for health problems, (c) the environment in which care is given, and (d) the end state of care, well-being. Yura and Torres (1975) then identified four overall themes based on a survey of 50 Bachelor of Science in Nursing (BSN) programs. They identified the following four concepts: (a) man, (b) health, (c) society, and (d) nursing.

Margaret Hardy, a noted nursing sociologist and philosopher from Boston University, was one of the first nurses to use the term *metaparadigm* in the nursing literature, published in *Advances in Nursing Science* in its inaugural year (1978). She described a metaparadigm as representing the broadest consensus within a discipline about its entities of interest and substantive focus. Then, in a *Journal of Nursing Scholarship* article, Jacqueline Fawcett (1984) drew from themes published earlier, and from her previous theoretical writings on central concepts of nursing, to formalize the nursing metaparadigm as comprising the four central concepts: person, health, environment, and nursing.

Given these four metaparadigm concepts, we can say that nursing ontology describes beliefs about the nature of human beings and health, the environment, and nursing practice. These concepts are not particularly helpful in guiding knowledge development until they are linked together and elaborated in various conceptual constructions, such as conceptual frameworks and metaparadigmatic statements. For example, Newman, Sime, and Corcoran-Perry (1991) put forth their metaparadigmatic statement: *Nursing is caring in the human health experience.* Historical and contemporary nursing theories and conceptual models are a rich source for learning about nursing ontology and the diversity of perspectives on the four metaparadigm concepts. As part of your philosophical inquiry in the substance of nursing, try developing your own metaparadigmatic statement of nursing.

Worldviews

A second way to understand or clarify your own nursing ontology is to examine the various worldviews used in nursing to frame perspectives about human beings and their health and health care practices. Nursing worldviews may also be called philosophies, discourses, or paradigms. They propose differing beliefs about human beings, health, practice, and other nursing concepts. Some regard worldviews or identification with any overarching perspective as a bias that can corrupt our thinking. Worldviews or Weltanschauung typically have been depicted as expressing an implicit, unexamined understanding about the world (Crotty, 1998). But everyone holds some kind of worldview. Articulating our worldviews and critically examining them with openness to other views is a useful process in knowledge development.

Worldviews, in fact, are applied widely across disciplines to understand systems from the cellular to individual to organizational levels. In nursing, worldviews range from mechanistic to developmental views of human health processes, from particularistic to holistic views of person–environment interactions, and from reactive to transformative views of human change. These frameworks originated in various disciplines and fields, including philosophy (e.g., Stephen Pepper's 1942 *World Hypotheses*), life-span developmental psychology (Lerner, 1986; Reed, 1995), complexity sciences (e.g., see biologist Stuart Kauffman, 1995, and Gaustello, Koopmans, & Pincus, 2009), and nursing (see Fawcett, 1993, for a succinct overview of extant nursing worldviews). Reflecting on your own beliefs and values and/or considering which, if any, worldviews align with your thinking is a form of philosophical inquiry. Doing this can help uncover areas of interest for research as well as expose biases that influence your path to knowledge development.

EPISTEMOLOGY

Epistemology refers to the study of the nature of knowledge, including what and how it is warranted as scientific knowledge in a discipline. Epistemological views have implications for selecting methods of theory development and research on the discipline's subject matter.

Several *patterns of knowing* are involved in producing nursing knowledge, for example, personal, practice, and ethical approaches with patients and families; empirical approaches that include scientific inquiry (Carper, 1978); sociopolitical approaches that inform nurses about sources of oppression in society and science (White, 1995); and emancipatory knowing that reveals injustices and why they endure, and what might be done to remove them (Chinn & Kramer, 2015).

Patterns of knowing may be used together to generate a theory. Alternatively, as Fawcett, Watson, Neuman, Walker, and Fitzpatrick (2001) suggested, each pattern may be used to generate a specific kind of theory, for example, empirical theory or ethical theory. Overall, nurses employ a diversity of research methods to obtain quantitative and qualitative data about the complex domain of nursing phenomena.

Epistemological views are also expressed in *philosophies of science*. These philosophies relate to how problems of study are conceptualized, and underlie methods of research and theory development.

PHILOSOPHY OF SCIENCE

So far we have traversed two paths: the outermost path (*philosophy of nursing*) and the innermost path (*theory*). The path to knowledge development is also influenced by *philosophy of science*, often from the discipline of philosophy. Philosophy of science is a field of study focused on the nature and practice of science, and the growth of scientific knowledge including the formulation, justification, and evaluation of scientific theories. The field consists of philosophies of science that propose differing beliefs about science and truth, knowledge and reality, mind and causality, and so on. And as with philosophy of nursing, philosophies of science more broadly frame our perspectives and methods in developing knowledge. So, exploring your own preferred philosophy of science along with the area of philosophical inquiry may give some insight into yourself in relation to your own journey along the path, like in what area you want to study or practice, and what research methods appeal to you.

Each research method generally is associated with a philosophical view or "methodology" underlying its characteristics. Major philosophies of science or "isms" that have influenced the practice of nursing science and knowledge development over the past century include positivism, postpositivism, constructionism, and postmodernism. Critical social theory is another philosophical perspective, and its major tenets, such as promoting awareness and emancipation from oppressive ideas and actions, may be integrated into research methods that derive from another philosophical view. For example, ethnography is associated with constructionism, but researchers may apply critical theory as well to use "critical ethnography" as their methodology. We conclude our walk on the philosophy of science portion of the path with an overview of several of these philosophical views in the next chapter.

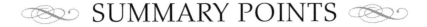

SUMMARY POINTS

1. The Spiral Path of Nursing Knowledge was designed to guide and encourage participation among nurses, particularly practicing nurses, in developing knowledge for the discipline.

2. The Path consists of six components: philosophy of nursing, philosophy of science, practice of science, practice of nursing, theoretical thinking, and theory.

3. Theory is a central component in the Path of Nursing Knowledge as the "vehicle of scientific knowledge."

4. Criteria for evaluation of scientific theory are based on both the traditional epistemic values of science and the social values of science and practice.

5. Questions about ontology, epistemology, and ethics are central issues in philosophical inquiry, relevant to many situations in nursing science and practice.

6. The metaparadigm and worldviews are aspects of ontology that provide philosophical bases for nursing theories and knowledge development.

7. Philosophy of science has several philosophies, sometimes referred to as "isms," that underlie the quantitative and qualitative methods used in research.

 # QUESTIONS FOR REFLECTION

1. What do you think about the practice of nursing being central in *developing*—not just *applying*—nursing knowledge? Do you develop new ideas from your practice experiences?

2. How do you envision your role in nursing knowledge—more as a consumer or a producer of nursing knowledge? Or both?

3. What theory are you familiar with through your studies in nursing or other disciplines?

4. Have you ever explored philosophical questions with your patients, friends, or family?

5. Reread Newman et al.'s (1991) "metaparadigmatic" statement and then try to compose your own brief statement: *"Nursing is. . . ."*

❧ REFERENCES ❧

Benner, P., Sutphen, M., Leonard, V., & Day, L. (2010). *Educating nurses: A call for radical transformation.* Stanford, CA: The Carnegie Foundations for the Advancement of Teaching.

Carper, B. (1978). Fundamental patterns of knowing in nursing. *Advances in Nursing Science, 1*(1), 13–23.

Chinn, P. L., & Kramer, M. K. (2015). *Knowledge development in nursing: Theory and process* (9th ed.). St. Louis, MO: Mosby.

Crotty, M. (1998). *The foundations of social research.* Thousand Oaks, CA: Sage.

Dubin, R. (1978). *Theory building* (Rev. ed.). New York, NY: The Free Press.

Eisner, E. (1985). *Learning and teaching the ways of knowing.* Chicago, IL: University of Chicago Press.

Fawcett, J. (1984). The metaparadigm of nursing: Present status and future refinements. *Image: The Journal of Nursing Scholarship, 16*(3), 84–87.

Fawcett, J. (1993). From a plethora of paradigms to parsimony in worldviews. *Nursing Science Quarterly, 6*, 56–58.

Fawcett, J., Watson, J., Neuman, B., Walker, P. H., & Fitzpatrick, J. J. (2001). On nursing theories and evidence. *Journal of Nursing Scholarship, 33*(2), 115–119.

Gaustello, S. J., Koopmans, J., & Pincus, D. (2009). *Chaos and complexity in psychology: The theory of nonlinear dynamical systems.* New York, NY: Cambridge University Press.

Hardy, M. E. (1978). Perspectives on nursing theory. *Advances in Nursing Science, 1*(1), 27–48.

Higgins, P. A., & Moore, S. M. (2000). Levels of theoretical thinking in nursing. *Nursing Outlook, 48*(4), 179–183.

Kauffman, S. (1995). *At home in the universe: The search of laws of self-organization and complexity.* New York, NY: Oxford University Press.

Kuhn, T. (1977). Objectivity, value judgment, and theory choice. In T. Kuhn (Ed.), *The essential tension: Selected studies in scientific tradition and change* (pp. 320–339). Chicago, IL: University of Chicago Press.

Latour, B. (1993). *We have never been modern* (C. Porter, Trans.). New York, NY: Harvester Wheatsheaf.

Lerner, R. M. (1986). *Concepts and theories of human development* (2nd ed.). New York, NY: Random House.

Lester, R. K., & Piore, M. J. (2004). *Innovation—The missing dimension.* Cambridge, MA: Harvard University Press.

Longino, H. E. (1990). *Science as social knowledge: Values and objectivity in scientific inquiry*. Princeton, NJ: Princeton University Press.

Longino, H. E. (1995). Gender, politics, and the theoretical virtues. *Synthese, 104*(3), 383–397.

Longino, H. E. (2002). *The fate of knowledge*. Princeton, NJ: Princeton University Press.

Longino, H. E. (2008). Values, heuristics, and the politics of knowledge. In M. Carrier, D. Howard, & J. Kourany (Eds.), *The challenge of the social and the pressure of practice: Science and value revisited* (pp. 68–86). Pittsburgh, PA: University of Pittsburgh Press.

McQueen, D. V. (2007). Critical issues in theory for health promotion. In D. V. McQueen & I. Kickbusch (Eds.), *Health and modernity: The role of theory in health promotion* (pp. 21–42). New York, NY: Springer.

Moore, K. D. (2010). *Wild comfort: The solace of nature*. Boston, MA: Trumpeter.

Newman, M. A., Sime, A. M., & Corcoran-Perry, S. A. (1991). The focus of the discipline of nursing. *Advances in Nursing Science, 14*(1), 1–6.

Peplau, H. E. (1952). *Interpersonal relations in nursing*. New York, NY: Putnam.

Pepper, S. P. (1942). *World hypotheses: A study in evidence*. Berkeley: University of California Press.

Reed, P. G. (1995). A treatise on nursing knowledge development for the 21st century: Beyond postmodernism. *Advances in Nursing Science, 17*(3), 70–84.

Reed, P. G. (1997). Nursing: The ontology of the discipline. *Nursing Science Quarterly, 10*(2), 76–79.

Reed, P. G. (2010). The spiral of nursing theory. *The Japanese Journal of Nursing Research, 4*(2), 87–92.

Rogers, M. E. (1970). *An introduction to the theoretical basis of nursing*. Philadelphia, PA: F. A. Davis.

Sibeon, R. (2007). An excursus in post-postmodern social science. In J. L. Powell & T. Owen (Eds.), *Reconstructing postmodernism: Critical debates* (pp. 29–40). New York, NY: Nova Science.

Smith, B. H. (2005). *Scandalous knowledge: Science, truth and the human*. Edinburgh, England: Edinburgh University Press.

Stehr, N. (Ed.). (2004). *The governance of knowledge*. New Brunswick, NJ: Transaction.

Suppe, F. (1977). *The structure of scientific theories* (2nd ed.). Chicago: University of Illinois Press.

Thomas, G. (2007). *Education and theory: Strangers in paradigms*. Berkshire, England: Open University Press.

Walker, L. O. (1971). Toward a clearer understanding of the concept of nursing theory. *Nursing Research, 20*, 428–435.

Weissman, D. (2008). *Styles of thought: Interpretation, inquiry, and imagination*. New York, NY: SUNY Press.

White, J. (1995). Patterns of knowing: Review, critique, and update. *Advances in Nursing Science, 17*(4), 73–86.

Yanchar, S., & Hill, J. R. (2003). What is psychology about? *Journal of Humanistic Psychology, 43*(1), 11–31.

Yura, H., & Torres, G. (1975). Today's conceptual framework within baccalaureate nursing programs. In National League for Nursing (Ed.), *Faculty-curriculum development, Part III: Conceptual Framework—Its meaning and function* (pp. 17–25). New York, NY: National League for Nursing.

2

A Philosophy of Nursing Science and Practice: Intermodernism

Pamela G. Reed

We pick up the spiral path where we left off in Chapter 1, reviewing several philosophical "isms" that are relevant to knowledge development in science as background to a discussion of *intermodernism,* my (emerging) philosophy of nursing science and nursing practice. Intermodernism evolved out of several years of studying philosophies of science and philosophical thinking about science and practice in nursing. We continue along the Path to consider how the *practice of science* and the *practice of nursing* are linked to knowledge development. The chapter concludes with a final turn to *theoretical thinking,* leaving you on the Path to carry on, using the theory tools of knowledge development you have picked up from this and subsequent chapters in the book for your own scholarly work.

A SHORT HISTORY OF SCIENCE

The path to knowledge changes over time as individuals, societies, and cultures change. And some historians suggest that we cannot say one perspective is better than another at achieving "truth." Understanding something about the history of science as it relates to your philosophy of nursing provides a context for you to clarify your own preferred philosophy of science.

From the 11th to 15th centuries, scientists (who were mostly astronomers) worked to align their observations with the accepted theory based on the aristotelian geocentric view of the universe (Oakley, 2000). Interestingly, science began by looking outward far away from Earth, and then worked inward toward human affairs (Magee, 2001). The path was mostly antiempirical and followed the methods of scholasticism; people did not study nature but instead employed logic, reason, and argument to understand and interpret the wisdom in the theology of the sacred texts and the philosophical views of the ancient Greeks such as Plato and Aristotle.

The key to modern science was a shift from testing ideas by argument and discussion to testing ideas by direct observations, measurement, and experimentation (Ferris, 2010; Losse, 2004). The aristotelian and religious worldviews of the Middle Ages gave way to the new scientific and heliocentric worldviews of the 16th century. The progression of modern science was fueled significantly by 17th century artisans working away with their own hands and ideas (Conner, 2005). Francis Bacon (1561–1626), mathematician and philosopher, is widely attributed with founding the scientific method that would launch modern science, but Conner (2005) reminds us that the evolution from earlier to modern approaches in knowledge development also occurred among the people in the daily practices of their work, generating indigenous knowledge that benefitted society.

A critical mass of thinkers occurred in the 18th century, building on the foundations of knowledge development from 17th century mathematicians and scientists as represented in the following events: the rationalism of Descartes, the scientific method and separation from metaphysics by Bacon, the abstractionism and mechanical discoveries about the universe by Newton, and the empiricism of John Locke. Knowledge was based on what could be "proved logically, tested scientifically, or verified empirically" (Ritchie, 2010, p. 3). This excluded other ways of knowing that derived from art, literature, religion, or personal insight. And it reinforced divisions between rationality and feeling, propositional truth and experience, verifiable history and personal meaning. Science during this time was built on the study of closed, physical systems, which were amenable to mathematical calculations, assumptions about invariant natural laws, and making precise predictions.

POSITIVISM

The scientific revolution of the 17th century helped foster 18th century enlightenment ideas about social progress, human reason, and intellectual freedom. Also during this time, positivism emerged as a philosophy of science in part through the demarcation of scientific discourse from other ways of knowing. It promised progress toward increasingly accurate causal explanations of the world and the unification of all scientific inquiry. This philosophy was based on an objectivist epistemology, which holds that meaning and reality exist independent of observers' values. Auguste Comte popularized the term *positivism* to distinguish knowledge that would come by speculation or reference to natural law as opposed to knowledge arrived at by direct experience. Comte and the members of the Vienna Circle held an interest in applying strictly empiricist methods of the natural sciences to the social and human sciences. They were interested not only in knowledge but also in precise methods to obtain knowledge. Additional emphases of logic, mathematics, and the use of language transformed raw positivism into logical positivism during the early 20th century.

General tenets of positivism include the following beliefs:

- Observation is objective and reveals facts, independent of culture and the observer.
- Mathematics and logic provide the form of theory.
- All of science can be reduced to physics.
- Scientific theories are or should be free of values.
- There is clear demarcation between science and all other ways of knowing, especially that concerning religion.
- Scientific knowledge is built as theories accumulate in a linear manner.
- The context of justification, not the context of discovery, is the more appropriate concern of science.

POSTPOSITIVISM

Twentieth-century discoveries led scientists to question some of their positivist assumptions. For example, during the 1920s, discoveries in physics about the structure of the atom and scientists' inability to determine the position of subatomic particles with accuracy stimulated questions about the nature of these particles, reality, and science. Scientists noted a gap between what they could directly verify by observation and the entities and concepts described in their theories—they had more theory than observable data! Their objects of study were too fast, too large, or too small to be directly observed (e.g., electromagnetism, gravity, evolution, embryo, and ego) and descriptions of these proposed entities required conceptual innovations.

Scientists began to realize that they were more actively constructing scientific knowledge than they were passively "receiving" it from nature above. The *received view*, coined by Hilary Putnam to describe the relationship between the reality and the objectivist scientist, was displaced by the *perceived view*, to acknowledge the role of perception in observing reality. Noted philosopher Karl Popper claimed that all observation takes place within the context of theory and is shaped by theory. Scientist and historian Thomas Kuhn (1962) put forth the idea that scientists in fact make sense of the world by looking through a conceptual apparatus called paradigms, which are based in history and change over time. By the 1960s, these and other influences weakened the dominance of objectivist epistemology, although vestiges still remain in science today, along with constructionist views of reality and knowledge. Thus, postpositivist scientists challenged and tempered the positivist claims of certitude and precise observations without negating its basic objectivist perspective of reality.

The following statements describe key tenets of postpositivism:

- Theory and data are not separable; theory influences perception of the "facts."
- Truth is based on achieving theories' correspondence with a reality that is observable yet cannot be fully known.
- Science produces inexact knowledge about reality.
- Scientific theories are underdetermined by observational evidence.
- Conjecture and deductive reasoning are used in theory development.
- Theories are tested by falsification, not verification.
- Scientific results are probabilistic.
- There are many paths (and methods) but only one truth, one reality.

CONSTRUCTIONISM

Constructionists hold an interpretive rather than objectivist view of truth and reality. They reject the view that there is objective truth and reality to be discovered. Meaning and knowledge are not discovered but rather are constructed through social interactions among individuals and between people and environment. Nevertheless, as one writer cogently pointed out, Kuhn's paradigm-shifting revolutions did not displace the discoveries made within the paradigm of scientific realism; space shuttles still fly according to Newton's laws (Ferris, 2010).

By *constructionism*, we understand knowledge to be a product of social processes between people and their environment (e.g., between researchers and participants, the nurse and the patient, the nursing discipline and society). Scientific theory involves interpretation and meaning-making from observations within a given context. Basic tenets of constructionism include the following ideas:

- Knowledge is a product of social interchanges and shared meanings.
- Truth is constructed, not discovered.
- Acceptable theories achieve coherence within a system of knowledge.
- Social, historical, and cultural factors are relevant in knowledge development.
- Scientists eschew foundational views but depend on shared ideas and values.
- Knowledge is built by consensus and shared meanings rather than by verification.

CRITICAL THEORY

Critical theory is a philosophical frame of reference for describing reality. It is related to an intellectual movement by social theorists of the Frankfurt School in the 1920s in response to the domination of positivist views and technological knowledge regarded as oppressing the working class (Bohman, 2016; Dant, 2003).

Critical theory, like the interpretive stance of constructionism, addresses social dimensions of knowledge development. But critical theory holds an additional ontological assumption that not all of reality is constructed; that is, real structural or social forces exist—independent of what we perceive or construct in our minds—that can constrain rationality and communication. Inquiry based on this philosophical view has a moral or normative aim in seeking to emancipate human beings from domination and oppression, beyond just describing or interpreting the data. Tenets of critical theory include the following views:

- Knowledge is influenced by language, power relations, and social processes that may convey oppressive ideologies.

- Theory necessarily acknowledges the role of social values and beliefs.

- Knowledge development includes methods of self-reflection, deconstruction, reflective practice, and critique of social structures and views that dominate and oppress human potential.

- A goal of critical theory is emancipation of self and others from dominating influences and various forms of oppression.

POSTMODERNISM

Popper and Kuhn's critiques of positivist science "somewhat unwittingly" laid the foundation for postmodernism (Ferris, 2010, p. 247). In postmodernism, science is regarded as a culturally influenced approach that is not necessarily any better than other forms of discourse (e.g., poetry and fiction) in conveying truths (Ferris, 2010, pp. 247–249). However, postmodernism resists description. Crotty (1998) applied the epistemological view of *subjectivism* to describe the postmodern stance as one where the inquirer imposes meaning on the data rather than constructs or elicits meaning out of the interaction. Not all postmodernists have this subjectivist view since they may be especially concerned with the detrimental effects that the inquiring or scientific gaze has on another.

Postmodernism cannot be summed up in a list of tenets. There are many differences across philosophical views. In general, however, postmodernists eschew four tenets found in either postpositivism or constructionism or both of these philosophies:

- Foundationalism—in *epistemology*, a belief in an unchanging foundation or in one view of truth

- Essentialism—in *metaphysics,* the view that people have an "essence"—characteristics that constitute universal features of human nature

- Realism—in *metaphysics,* the belief in a reality that exists independent of mind or the historical or social context

- Representationalism—in *philosophy of language,* the view that neither a scientist nor an artist can reproduce or "mirror" reality. Postmodernists may employ a method called *deconstruction* (from poststructuralism) to reveal the "foolishness" of modern science attempts to represent reality through research findings.

Postmodernism's iconoclastic and pluralistic attitudes opened up new possibilities for nursing knowledge development (Reed, 1995). This philosophy of science helped dislodge nurses from dichotomous thinking about science and art, qualitative and quantitative data, empirical and spiritual, facts and values, and theory and practice. This process is not unlike the interpretive method of the hermeneutic circle, where one spirals back and forth between dichotomous or contradictory elements (e.g., part and whole, what is understood and what is not understood, illness and wellness) to gain better understanding of a concept or situation. Nurses entertain the possibility of multiple interpretations, meanings, and methods in knowledge development.

Importantly, like all scientists of modern philosophical views, postmodernists share a value for skepticism; an enthusiasm for discovery; and a desire for emancipation from ignorance, prejudice, and oppressive authority. Judd (2009) explains that even Bacon (1561–1626), philosopher and founder of the modern scientific method, was an exemplary model for breaking the rules in the interest of knowledge development. Bacon's empirical method and spirit of experimentation separated him from the beliefs of medieval church scholars and Aristotle's principles of natural philosophy to inspire liberal intellectual thinking in a new practice of science.

INTERMODERNISM: A PLACE BETWEEN *MODERNISMS*

As we travel around the Path from philosophy of nursing and philosophy of science, let us stop just before the next turn where *philosophy* transitions into *action* with the practice of nursing, to consider one final philosophical perspective as it relates to our efforts in knowledge development. The postmodern discourse on science may have led you to question the value of traditional scientific approaches in knowledge development, if not to construe science itself as a hegemonic practice incongruent with nursing's humanistic values. However, the use of reason, questioning, and skepticism that drove the scientific revolution of the 17th century is still valued today and nursing is very much a scientific discipline. Science endures today as a critical, open, and reflective practice that generates knowledge for a discipline. So I suggest that we extend our thinking to clarify a philosophical stance *between* modernisms—between modern and postmodern views—that may better fit 21st century nursing and support practices of nursing science not represented by the other perspectives individually. I have named this new perspective *intermodernism*.

Intermodernism builds on an initial formulation of a philosophy of nursing science called *neomodernism* that I presented several years ago (Reed, 1995, 2006); some have since applied this perspective to advanced practice, science, and research (e.g., Anderson & Whall, 2011; Arslanian-Engoren, Hicks, Whall, & Algase, 2005; Burns, 2014; Liehr & Smith, 2007; Whall & Hicks, 2002).

Intermodernism is a heterodox philosophy of science in that it departs somewhat from traditional views yet finds wisdom in existing philosophies. The term *intermodernism* indicates an approach that does not abandon useful categories of science yet creates a space for us to think about what features we would like or need in a philosophy of science to facilitate knowledge development through our practices of science and nursing care.

Intermodernism is reflected in the overall structure of the spiral path as well as in each element in the path. This is depicted by the arrow in Figure 2.1. The entire

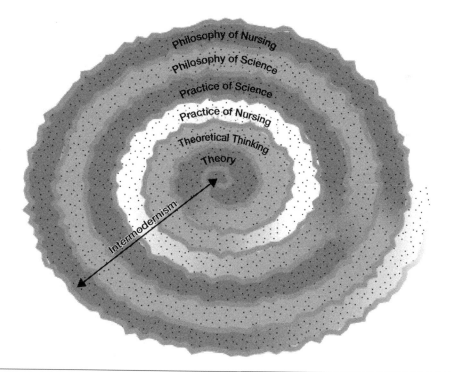

FIGURE 2.1 Intermodernism and the spiral path of nursing knowledge development.

knowledge process represented by the spiral path—the nonlinear, nonhierarchical arrangement of elements; the absence of an end point and the openness of theorizing; and the distinct yet merged areas of practice, science, and theory—all emanate from an intermodern view of knowledge development.

The intermodern path accounts for various contingencies that postmodernists informed us about in our search for truth, the unavoidable influences on our theorizing and knowledge development. The turns of the Path represent a number of these—for example, personal beliefs; life experiences; socioeconomic and political factors; and professional experiences, expertise, and worldview—and are regarded as opportunities that enrich rather than constrain knowledge.

THE MIDDLE WAY

Intermodernism describes a new philosophy of nursing science and practice, but it does not veer too far off the familiar path of science and knowledge development. It honors the wisdom of the middle way. Intermodernism bridges the limitations of a strictly modern view and a strictly postmodern view of knowledge and science. There is an increasing number of scholars from various disciplines attempting to bridge modernism and postmodernism, to broaden approaches to knowledge development beyond boundaries of postpositivism but without the nihilism or other limitations of postmodernism (e.g., Mouzelis, 2008). These disciplines include biology, economics, fine arts, literature, psychology, and several health care fields such as health promotion and occupational therapy. Intermodernism shares with postmodernism and modernism an enthusiasm for discovery balanced by healthy skepticism and appreciation for the mystery in life, and the aim of emancipation from ignorance, prejudice, domination, and oppressive authority.

The intermodern view maintains a focus on the person (and other living systems or organizations) as having innate value, emotional and moral senses, and other internal attributes, yet acknowledges the reality of contextual influences (e.g., historical, political, sociocultural) on individuals, families, and communities.

Intermodernism is similar to post-postmodern views, which preserve strands of stability while avoiding radical extremes (Hickman, 2007). Post-postmodernists "tend to be interested in political philosophy, taking democracy and its ideals as a model for addressing philosophical issues." They are pluralist in outlook, but also value "disciplinary structure in scholarship. Fields such as epistemology, theology, philosophy of science, and the history of ideas," which were marginalized by postmodernism, have gained renewed interest by post-postmodernism (*Concise Routledge Encyclopedia of Philosophy*, 2000, pp. 700–701).

The middle way is pluralistic, encouraging a diversity of ideas. Intermodernism avoids some of the extremes in postmodern philosophy found, for example, in Kuhn's *revolutions* and Foucault's *ruptures* (Smith, 2005). Through paradoxical rather than dialectical thinking, differences in theories and methods can coexist without being resolved into one synthesis. Instead of the Kuhnian perspective that paradigms are incommensurable and therefore logically must compete through revolution for scientific progress to occur (Stepin, 2005), pluralism allows for new thinking; different paradigms and theories can coexist and still undergo change without being integrated or subsumed into one right view.

However, intermodernists do not confuse *pluralism* with *relativism* because they identify with some shared values in their science community and commit to a common paradigm to facilitate knowledge development, if even within the nurse's particular practice or academic community. Shared values, for example, are personal autonomy, self-development, agency, humanism, emancipation, and justice.

PATTERN IN THE UNIVERSE

Intermodernism affirms a perception or belief in an underlying order in our local universe. The universe is "dappled" with patterns, where "laws that describe this world are a patchwork, not a pyramid" (Cartwright, 1999). Within an intermodern view, scientific inquiry and practice are based, in part, on the idea that laws, tendencies, or patterns exist in the phenomena of interest insofar as our theories inform us. Scientific progress is related to the extent that a discipline's theories describe and explain these phenomena and help solve conceptual and practical problems. It is a pragmatic more than an objectivist view of reality and truth.

Moreover, Carter and New (2004) suggested that the positivist's aim to discover universal laws has been exaggerated since many of the laws are not invariant but rather refer to "tendencies" or probabilities that events will occur according to a given principle. Cartwright (1999) proposes a view of reality that is appealing to intermodernism in nursing (with its focus on understanding health processes in human–environment interactions) in her philosophical view that science depends on knowledge of capacities, not on our knowledge of laws.

> *Our most wide-ranging scientific knowledge is not knowledge of laws but knowledge of the natures of things, knowledge that allows us to build nomological machines never before seen giving rise to new laws never before dreamt of* (Cartwright, 1999, p. 4).

The following are 11 tenets of the intermodern perspective:

- *In-between-ness:* Theorists work in-between modernism and postmodernism, between extremes and contradictions, yet somehow outside of traditional methods. Thinking can be "[r]adical without being revolutionary, eccentric without being trivial" and is valued for its "departure from 'high' modernism . . . ." (Bluemel, 2004, p. 66).

- *Nursing:* Acknowledges modernist descriptions of nursing as a practice and a scientific body of knowledge, but also defines nursing ontologically as inherent processes of well-being within and among human systems (Reed, 1997). Understandings of nursing go beyond modernist descriptions that separate the practice of science from the practice of nursing care to conceptualize nursing as a process that may occur (a) externally through the actions and interactions of nurses to facilitate well-being or (b) intrapersonally and even internally where, for example, psychosocial and biological processes engage the person's inner resources for well-being.

- *Truth:* Truth is defined neither by theories' *correspondence* with one source of truth nor necessarily by theories' *coherence* with a cluster of other theories, but through the *coordination* of multiple theoretical ideas focused on addressing a similar problem. In addition, local truths are valued but an external "corrective" or paradigm is regarded as useful in determining just what is emancipating, good, healthful, and other value-laden truths used in nursing. Even this source of truth though is not a universal truth; it is truth as found in our theories and paradigms.

- *Empiricism:* A new empiricism based on a broadened perspective of what comprises nursing evidence. It is not objectivist but includes both objective and subjective data, and valorizes the perspectives of patients and families as central in the discovery and justification of knowledge. In addition, there is a network of human, nonhuman, technological, and hybrid elements that informs knowledge development (Latour & Woolgar, 1986).

- *Reality:* Reality is found neither "out there" independent of the thinker (realist) nor completely within the thinker's mind (idealist). Both realist and antirealist. Reality emerges and acquires its specificity, for example, *through* the nurse's theories, interactions, and actions in health care. Acknowledges an underlying pattern in terms of what is described in theories.

- *Methods:* Systematic methods are important to the scientific enterprise, but it is also recognized that science is a messy process, a "mangle of practice" (Pickering, 2005), a fact illuminated by the field of science studies. Knowledge development in nursing practice then exemplifies both the systematic and messy nature of science.

- *Openness:* Being open to critique, self-correction, and change and an ongoing reflection on one's theory and practice are essential in knowledge development. Openness is congruent with the open, self-organizing nature of human systems in process with their environments.

- *Discovery:* The context of discovery—the dynamic situations and influences under which knowledge is created—achieves an importance much greater than it had in modern science, which focused on the context of justification of theories. Discovery involves multiple ways of knowing that inform and extend empirical knowing. *Abductive reasoning*, which is more than the mere combination of inductive and deductive logic, is a dominant pattern of scientists and practitioners. Scientific "findings" are constructed more than discovered, but they are "neither arbitrary nor are they constructed out of nothing" (Hickman, 2007, p. 28).

- *Epistemology:* This promotes an expanded epistemology in which science and practice partner to create knowledge. There is a reimagining of theory in relation to practice as a *source* not just as a *repository* of knowledge. Practice is a pattern of knowing that informs empirical knowing and knowledge development. Knowledge development is pragmatic and performative, found in experience and in the doing, as well as in thinking and in the reflecting. Technology provides new tools, instruments, equipment, machines, biotechnology, and other means for observing the unobservable, for facilitating wholeness in a posthuman culture, and for generating knowledge (and including "thing knowledge"; see Baird, 2004; Locsin, 2009) about nursing processes that promote well-being.

- *Romanticism:* This recognizes the reality of the human quest for meaning, goodness, and beauty. Metaphysical views are included in what are considered focuses for empirical study and theorizing in nursing. Spirituality and purpose in life, for example, can be studied empirically as expressions of human experiences related to well-being. It embraces both the scientific view and belief in an abiding mystery in what can be known (Raymo, 2008; Tauber, 2009). Nonepistemic (social, cultural, emotional) as well as epistemic (cognitive, logic) values are relevant in scientific inquiry. Human beings and indeed the universe are simply too complex and broad to be fully understood by commonsense observation or objectivist scientific study.

- *Nightingale:* This scientist and scholarly practitioner is a symbol to remind us to strive for the following events: (a) reclaim the health and unitary focus of person–environment and inner healing capacity espoused by Nightingale; (b) value and build upon nursing's indigenous knowledge, found in classic theorists and scholars, and in lay persons in their everyday health experiences; (c) decolonize our discipline of other health care practices and paradigms that rob nurses of opportunities to build knowledge and provide care from a nursing perspective of health, illness, and end of life.

This list of tenets of intermodernism is incomplete and open. You may think of other potential tenets as you continue to read and reflect. In the following sections, notice the presence of this philosophical perspective. There are other examples of intermodernism in knowledge development throughout other chapters as well. Intermodern ideas permeate this book.

THE PRACTICE OF SCIENCE

The practice of science refers to the systematic methods and strategies of knowledge development used in theoretical and empirical research. The practice of science in the context of nursing care can generate knowledge and theories that are especially relevant and timely for practice. (See Chapter 11 on practice-based evidence research for a discussion of this idea.) Various research methods are available that can be applied or modified and refined for practice-based research. Regardless of the method used, it is understood that no data are "raw" in the modern sense, as direct indicators of reality, pure and devoid of influences. More realistically, science is a mangle of social processes (Pickering, 2005); scientific discovery is not one "aha" moment, but involves an ongoing cycle of theory generation, evaluation, and revision (Darden, 2009).

NURSES, ENGINEERS, AND INNOVATION

In 20th century nursing, science was modern, or so it seemed, and nurses were instructed to maintain a separation between roles as clinicians and researchers. Nurse scientists did the research and developed the knowledge that was then handed down to the clinician to apply in practice. However, as Latour (1993) explained, *we have never been modern*. We have never completely separated research from the values and experiences in practice. Rigid separation between the practice and science of nursing is untenable today. Knowledge development in nursing brings scientific inquiry and nursing practice together more closely where nurses' observations and interactions with people in health-related situations provide opportunities for knowledge development, testing, and evaluation. Knowledge need not be handed down when it is generated in practice.

In elaborating on the innovative thinking of engineers, Petroski (2010) provides a description of the engineer that can be applied to the nurse scholar in practice: It is the engineer's ability not just for the "observational and predictive thinking" used in traditional science, but for "conceptual and constructive thinking" that creates new knowledge in the context of engineering problems (p. 15). The innovative and original knowledge of engineers that Petroski (2010) champions reaches beyond the translation or application of knowledge produced by the bench science of physicist or chemist. The knowledge developed by the engineer "cannot be taken off nature's shelf; they are *pure creations* of engineering" (author's emphasis, Petroski, 2010, p. 22).

The relationship between the practice of science and the practice of nursing care can foster new knowledge out of the pragmatics and problems of practice. As Petroski (2010) further explained, "Pure science and pure truth are things of the past." Science is no longer "unfettered by practical concerns" free to pursue natural phenomena not connected to practice (p. 114). He witnessed reversal of the linear model of R&D (Research and Development) to D&R where the emphasis is on "real-world directed research" (p. 118).

The practice of science typically employs two sets of tools: theory and research. Theoretical ideas inspire and guide the research, but it is the practice of nursing that actually motivates knowledge development.

THE PRACTICE OF NURSING

In looking at the spiral path, you will notice that there is no clear demarcation between the practice of science and the practice of nursing. This is the reality of practice-based knowledge development. The practice of nursing is a *science and an art* of combining the contingencies of the moment, including diverse patterns of knowing, with systematic and scientific knowledge to create a caregiving situation. Similarly, Georgia O'Keeffe created her works of art from an inner creative vision but also knew the science of her practice, that is, the technical skills, methods, and basic theoretical concepts of composition, balance, and color.

The practice of nursing is also a *theoretical endeavor*. A central thesis of this chapter is that theory can emerge out of the practice of nursing and nurses' caregiving situations. With ample reflection on and in practice situations coupled with a fund of clinical knowledge and some understanding of theories and theory development, nurses may produce compelling theoretical knowledge. However, this thesis requires more inquiry. As Clarke, James, and Kelly (1996) explained many years ago, "Theory is created at the moment of action through a complex, and as yet inadequately understood, process of reflecting in action" (p. 176).

A few scholars have taken on the challenge of explaining practice-based science and practice-based theory development, creatively extending Dickoff and James's (1968) classic thesis on "practice theory" (e.g., Diers, 1995/2004; Doane, Browne, Reimer, MacLeod, & MacLellan, 2009; Doane & Varcoe, 2005; Kim, 1993, 1999). But one scholar in particular addressed more fully the question as to how nursing theory and nursing knowledge are generated in practice—Hildegard Peplau. And she did this decades before others. She published most of her theoretical ideas during the modern era of nursing, but her thinking was intermodern. Peplau's cycle of inquiry refutes any modern approach to theory that dichotomizes knowledge production and application.

TRANSFORMING PRACTICE KNOWLEDGE INTO NURSING KNOWLEDGE

Although practice is an undertheorized context for knowledge development, Peplau's (1952, 1988) classic works provide excellent insights into how knowledge and theory may be generated in practice. Peplau was known for her theory on the interpersonal relations published in 1952. However, what many nurses do not know of Peplau is her *cycle of inquiry* whereby she described practice as a process of transforming practice knowledge into nursing knowledge.

Peplau presented the nurse–patient relationship as a context for conceptual innovations. Her strategy for practice-based inquiry has some similarity to that described in Neurath's boat image. Otto Neurath was a philosopher of science who likened theory building to the rebuilding of a ship at sea:

> *We are like sailors who have to rebuild their ship on the open sea, without ever being able to dismantle it in drydock and reconstruct it from the best components.* (Neurath, 1983, p. 92)

A key aspect of the approach is building on existing knowledge and theories while bringing in new ideas from clinical experiences for the innovation of concepts for theory development. Existing theories provide a base for developing and evaluating new ideas. Knowledge builds on itself.

Peplau's Cycle of Inquiry[1]

Nursing practice typically has been viewed as a context for *applying* but not *developing* knowledge, but the therapeutic relationships that are integral to nursing practice are also a means for testing and building theory. Peplau's work elevated nursing practice to the level of scholarship; that is, she connected nurse–patient interactions to theoretical ideas and concepts. She synthesized ideas from theories of Harry Stack Sullivan, Abraham Maslow, and Erich Fromm. Yet her approach to inquiry for nursing let the patient and the "voice of nursing" (Johnson, 1993) be heard above the theory. In doing this, Peplau introduced an approach to knowledge development that was anchored in nursing practice and in the science and art of the nurse–patient interaction. Development and testing of explanations through the interpersonal process between the patient and the nurse were done for therapeutic purposes—but, according to Peplau, this interpersonal process was also a strategy for generating nursing knowledge. Steps 1, 2, and 3 describe her strategy of transforming practice knowledge into nursing knowledge. These steps are an early example of *abductive thinking* in developing nursing knowledge.

STEP 1: OBSERVATION OF FUNDAMENTAL UNITS. Knowledge development, according to Peplau, begins with observations made in the context of practice. For Peplau, this context was primarily the nurse–patient relationship. Observation preceded conceptual interpretations. Peplau (1952) outlined various methods of observation that yielded knowledge, including spectator observation, role-playing, and random observation. However, Peplau (1952, 1992a) emphasized participant observation, in which a nurse uses self as both the instrument and object of observation while participating in the interpersonal process with a patient.

According to Peplau, a nurse enters a situation with theoretical understanding, personal bias, and previously acquired nursing knowledge. Patients enter with their

---

1. Portions of this text were adapted from Reed (1996) Transforming practice knowledge into nursing knowledge—A revisionist analysis of Peplau. *Image: Journal of Nursing Scholarship, 28*(1), 29–33. Reprinted with permission from John Wiley & Sons.

knowledge and with the powers and capabilities of a developing human being. Patients possess the principal data for inquiry in the form of underdeveloped or unused competencies, subconscious meanings, and personal knowledge. Nurses possess knowledge of methods to help patients make use of their competencies and to regain well-being.

Peplau (1992b) explained that, while on a "philosophical level" human beings may not be reducible, elements about human beings can be studied and measured to develop nursing knowledge at the "theoretical level" (p. 88). Scientists and scholars agree that knowledge production, at least in part, involves placing boundaries around phenomena. Relevant "units of observation" according to Peplau are those that are meaningful and useful to patients, measurable, and definable, and that can be replicated and compared with other data (Peplau, 1952, p. 270). Fundamental units of inquiry within Peplau's theory (1952, 1988) are *processes* and *patterns* and the *problems* that can emerge from them.

Processes refer to behaviors that develop over time in observable phases (Peplau, 1987, 1992a). She included nursing therapeutic processes, such as the four-phased interpersonal relationship, as that which "co-operates with and assists" other processes to move the patient toward health (p. 125).

Patterns comprise separate thoughts, feelings, or actions that share the same theme or aim (Peplau, 1987, 1992a). Patterns that are shared by two or more people are called "pattern integrations," and they may be mutual (when both parties exhibit the same set of behaviors), complementary, or antagonistic.

Thus, building knowledge entails observation of human processes and patterns, fundamental units of study. The *problems* that arise from these may also be studied, while drawing from knowledge about the underlying processes and patterns to produce theoretical explanations.

STEP 2: PEELING OUT AND TESTING THEORETICAL EXPLANATIONS: PEPLAU'S ABDUCTIVE APPROACH. Once initial observations are made by a nurse in an interpersonal relationship, theoretical concepts are then "peeled out" and drawn into the interpersonal process to explain observed phenomena (Letter to Geraldine Ellis cited in Welt & O'Toole, 1989; Peplau, 1988). This process is not unlike abductive reasoning described in the section Theoretical Thinking. *Peeling out* refers to abstracting concepts from clinical knowledge and from existing scientific theories and conceptual frameworks; these concepts represent the phenomena observed in practice, and are subsequently connected together in a logical way to formulate a conceptual or theoretical framework. Peplau (1988) identified this as part of a nursing process of "interpreting observations." This process includes such investigative activities as creative invention, decoding, subdividing data, categorizing data, identifying layers of meaning at different levels of abstraction, and applying a conceptual framework to explain phenomena.

Through "peeling out," hypotheses are drawn from the nurse's observations (Peplau, 1952, p. 269). These tentative explanations that are formulated are then validated with the patient and tested for their meaningfulness and usefulness in the context of the nurse–patient relationship.

Peplau's theorizing was not limited by a strict adherence to formulating operational definitions or deducing testable statements from existing "high theories." Rather, Peplau's regard for universal patterns in psychosocial development, learning, and other human experiences was tempered by her emphasis on the clinically based reality created during encounters with patients (Reed, 1996).

STEP 3: TRANSFORMING ENERGY AND TRANSFORMING KNOWL-EDGE. The final step is application of theoretical knowledge through interactions with patients. This results in the transformation of practice knowledge into nursing knowledge. The term *application* hardly captures this transformation, because it requires aesthetic perspective, intellectual competencies, and clinical judgment (Peplau, 1988, p. 13).

The test of the truthfulness of knowledge, according to Peplau (1952, 1988), was not based on how well the knowledge corresponded to a preexisting theory but how effective it was in helping patients enhance their self-understanding and developmental progress. [Notice her pragmatic rather than objectivist aim.] Nursing knowledge is developed in the context of practice through synthesis of (a) existing scientific theories, clinical observation, and judgment of nurses, and (b) knowledge and active participation of the patients. Thus, Peplau's interpersonal process provides a context for engaging in both nursing care (helping the patient transform anxiety into productive energy) and nursing science (peeling out theories, testing them, and, in so doing, transforming practice into nursing knowledge.)

NURSING KNOWLEDGE

In Peplau's (1952) cycle of inquiry, nursing knowledge that is generated through nursing practice is further evaluated and refined through research methods. The resulting knowledge becomes part of a practicing nurse's repertoire of nursing knowledge, which undergoes transformation and validation in subsequent nurse–patient encounters, as the cycle of inquiry begins again.

During the early modern era of nursing, nursing researchers often borrowed knowledge from other disciplines to be passed on to the practitioners. However, Peplau's (1952) cycle of inquiry produced practice-based nursing knowledge rather than borrowed knowledge. It is *nursing* knowledge by virtue of its link to nursing processes and nursing practice. In sum, Peplau's cycle of inquiry provides a classic yet progressive perspective on the central thesis of this chapter: *Nursing practice is more than a context for applying a tested and refined theory: Practice is a context for initiating and testing theory.*

THEORETICAL THINKING

Theoretical thinking, identified near the center of the figure, spirals through the entire journey of the Path. All disciplines by definition have theories and scientists engage in theoretical thinking. In fact, everyone has working theories about how they view their world and how things function. Children create their own theories to explain how and why things occur. Adolescents and adults do this as well. Practitioners think theoretically to make sense of their everyday encounters. It is the scientists who are unusual in regard to theorizing—they have explicit rules about how to develop theories, how to use them, and how to judge their theories.

Theoretical thinking is the basis of our humanity. It is in our ability to "make theories, to test them from experience, and then make new and better ones, that intelligence emerges" (Gopnik, 2009, p. 186). Gopnik explained that the scientist's ability to theorize reflects a person's ability to continue to learn, to be open to new thinking, and to define the world in new ways. This ability, he says, brings dignity to those who make theories.

All thinking is impregnated with theory, especially our scientific conceptualizations. Ferris (2010) explained that we are now so enlightened about the presence of theory that we tend to mock the 17th century idea that science is merely the sum of observations and take for granted our realization that facts and observations are theory laden. Gopnik (2009), in his publication about Darwin's work, explained that

"it is in the jump beyond, to a general rule, a theory, even a vision, that science advances." (p. 71)

ABDUCTIVE REASONING

Theoretical thinking in nursing, and particularly nursing practice, may be described largely by the process of *abduction*. Abduction was first described by philosopher of science Charles Peirce (1934) and then elaborated by Hanson (1958) to propose a form of reasoning involved in discovering a plausible explanation, inferring a hypothesis, or generating a theory. This form of reasoning is the third but most important form of logic, next to inductive and deductive logic. Abduction generates more substantial knowledge than can either deduction or induction alone.

With abduction, the theorist brings together observation and theory, experiences, and existing knowledge, to posit a potential explanation for a given situation or event. The nurse takes a creative, conceptual leap to posit possible reasons or underlying processes to explain its occurrence. This explanation may extend beyond what is readily observed at the present time. The abduction creates a holding place for evidence found later to better explain the underlying process (Weissman, 2008).

Nurses characteristically mistake their abductive reasoning for intuition. Nurses in practice often must act upon their best judgment in the absence of perfect knowledge by making simultaneous connections between their observations and interactions with patients and extant theories and other patterns of knowing. Better understanding of this expertise for theoretical thinking may enable nurses to more deliberately produce theoretical knowledge out of their practice encounters.

Abductive reasoning produces open theories. The practitioner uses new data and ideas as they arise to test and modify or refine the theory. There are several sources in the literature that outline examples, details, and steps in abductive thinking (e.g., Montgomery, 2006; Råholm, 2010; Weissman, 2008), although most focus on knowledge development by the researcher rather than the practitioner. Nevertheless, it is likely to be the new generation of doctoral nurses who will better describe abductive thinking for knowledge development by practicing nurses.

CHAMPIONING THEORETICAL THINKING IN PRACTICE

For nurses in particular, theoretical thinking provides the disciplinary focus and basis of our practice. And theorizing helps nurses understand the clinical phenomena with which they deal every day. By theorizing, nurses create a mental image of a concept or an event—to see, to ponder, to understand, and to communicate with others—and then use in practice in some therapeutic or meaningful way (Thorne, 2005). By theorizing, practitioners make sense of their daily lives.

Disciplines share knowledge and borrow theories from other disciplines. However, the strength of a profession's jurisdiction in practice and the clarity of a discipline's identity and contribution to society are dependent on the explication of a discipline's own theories (Abbott, 1988; Potvin & Balbo, 2007). A sustaining characteristic of both a science and a profession is having theories that are unique to that discipline. More specifically, the mark of scholarship in nursing practice is not the practice alone but when "the intellectual work [of the nurse] . . . raises the clinical instance to the level of theory" (Diers, 1995/2004, p. 84). Both the conceptual and the empirical are valued.

Theories have important functions in a practice. Kurt Lewin (1951) is often quoted as saying, "there is nothing as practical as a good theory" (p. 169). Theoretical thinking moves knowledge forward by imagining new concepts and mechanisms occurring in practice. "It is in the leap of the data, not the heap of the data . . . [where] the advance lies" (Gopnik, 2009, p. 71). Knowledge developed in the form of theory does not merely describe a situation or concepts in isolation; it links concepts, ideas, and events to each other to propose some underlying process.

The contemporary writer bell hooks's (1999) description of writing relates to theorizing in practice: We do it "to find secrets in experience that are obscured from ordinary sight: to uncover hidden coherences in what seems to be a mere jumble of unrelated events and details, and to find incoherence in what appears to be strictly ordered; to make transparent what is opaque, and to expose opacity in what seems transparent" (p. 40).

So, theories give us new perspectives, sensitize us to what patients are saying, and help us listen in new ways and discover new ideas that can be of greater help to patients. And when our theories cannot fully explain, they can offer up abstract concepts, as a place holder for things we cannot quite grasp while we forge ahead in knowledge development, rebuilding our ship as we sail the sea.

Theoretical thinking in nursing reflects the middle way of intermodernism in that it involves analysis and interpretation, systematic thought and imagination. Theorizing is not the result of simply employing analytical thinking and a logical, standardized procedure. Nor is it a process of unplanned flashes of insight (Meheus & Nickles, 2009). It takes a little of both, plus adequate doses of creativity, imagination, and perseverance. Theories help us avoid errors from two extremes, of narrow empiricism that limits our sights to one way of knowing and the extreme of "unanchored abstract thought" that attempts to explain all (McQueen, 2007, p. 22).

SUSTAINING DISCIPLINARY KNOWLEDGE: LINKING PRACTICE AND THEORY

Van den Daele (2004) explained that since the 19th century, modern science progressed as the "implicit and embodied knowledge of the practitioner [was replaced] by the explicit and disembodied knowledge of the scientists" (p. 34). However, he goes on to warn that the traditional scientists' vision for knowledge development may be too narrow for the increasingly complex nature of society. "In dealing with complexity, the limits of the *knowing scientists* may be narrower than the limits of the *knowing practitioner*, for instance in handling human life and behavior, organizations, or technical systems" (p. 34). Clearly, the wisdom of the practitioner along with other nurses will be needed to build the knowledge and theories of the 21st century.

According to 20th century modernist practices of science, nursing research and practice were regarded as separate domains: Scientific knowledge was developed by the researchers and then handed over to practicing nurses through mechanisms variously called dissemination, application, translation, or research utilization to practicing nurses. Postmodernist ideas of the later third of the 20th century challenged traditional thinking across many disciplines about knowledge generation. The movement stimulated new ideas about the relationship between theory and practice and about who should participate in defining truth for a discipline. Shifts in thinking about knowledge development and practice are still unfolding. During the 21st century, intermodernism, as a philosophy of nursing science and practice, may provide some guidance and inspiration along the way.

As a discipline rich with practice, theory, and research dimensions, nurses can be leaders in theory innovations that advance societal welfare. Nursing science and practice employ multiple patterns of knowing while still valuing certain foundational principles first expressed in the grand theories. Classic nursing theories are still appreciated for their historical significance in distinguishing nursing among other health care disciplines and as a theory foundation for knowledge development, but new ideas about theory and knowledge development are on the horizon—ideas generated by the knowledge potential inherent in the burgeoning of doctoral nurses who will enter practice as well as academe and other positions in the next decade. Nursing theories will have to be accessible, flexible, and responsive to the knowledge needs of practicing nurses and the public. Theory will not so much be applied or disseminated from research to practice as it will emerge from scholarly thinking in practice, and then continue to be transformed as practice contexts change.

Theories are windows for the world to peer into the knowledge of disciplines. *What knowledge will enter the world through nursing?* Nursing has an increasing number of doctoral level practicing nurses who will become an untapped resource for knowledge development if they are not educated on processes of theory innovation as well as research. Historians of science tell us emphatically that to sustain our profession, *knowledge must become disciplinary*; that is, there must be an ongoing and organized core of like-minded individuals who work together in building knowledge into useful and meaningful theories of that discipline. Our large and complex discipline needs a network of strategies and a network of scholars for knowledge.

Knowledge development draws from philosophical, empirical, and theoretical dimensions of nursing knowledge. A scholar sees all practices as inquiry, always asking why, yet appreciating the mystery, and always reaching for new ideas—whether predominantly as a practitioner, philosopher, scientist, theorist, teacher, or learner. We need nursing scholars in all practices who can walk the path of inquiry to build nursing knowledge. Engaging and educating practicing nurses more deliberately, along with other graduate nurses, in theory innovations will provide nursing with a more sustainable approach to fostering development of knowledge for our future health care needs.

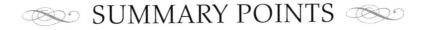 SUMMARY POINTS

1. The history of science has produced several philosophical perspectives (positivism, postpositivism, constructionism, critical theory, postmodernism) that influence knowledge development in science.

2. Intermodernism is a philosophy of nursing science and practice that sits between modernism and postmodernism, combining selected key elements of both and presenting new ideas about nursing knowledge and theory development.

3. The practice of science refers to the systematic methods and strategies of knowledge development used in theoretical and empirical research. The practice of science in the context of nursing care can generate knowledge and theories that are especially relevant and timely for practice.

4. The practice of nursing is an art, a science, and also a theoretical endeavor.

5. A central thesis of this chapter is that theory can emerge out of the practice of nursing and nurses' caregiving situations. It is not yet clear how nurses generate knowledge and theory in practice, although some scholars have written about this process.

6. Peplau's cycle of inquiry provides a classic yet progressive perspective on nursing practice as more than a context for applying a tested and refined theory: Practice is a context for initiating and testing theory.

7. Theoretical thinking in nursing, and particularly nursing practice, may be described largely by the process of *abduction*. Abduction was first described by philosopher of science Charles Peirce (1934).

8. A sustaining characteristic of both a science and a profession is having theories that are unique to that discipline.

 QUESTIONS FOR REFLECTION

1. How has this chapter helped you answer the question as to how knowledge (or theory) is generated in nursing practice?

2. Which philosophical view or ism was most meaningful or useful to you at this time in your career?

3. What component(s) of the Path were most helpful in understanding how nursing knowledge can be developed? Which components of the path left you with questions?

4. Eleven tenets of intermodernism were proposed. What is another that you might add beside one of the letters? How closely do you identify with the perspectives of this new philosophical view? Do you disagree with some tenets?

5. How has this chapter helped you begin to think about your own theory innovations through your nursing practice or research?

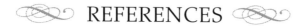 REFERENCES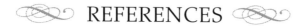

Abbott, A. (1988). *The system of professions.* Chicago, IL: University of Chicago Press.

Anderson, C. A., & Whall, A. L. (2011). A philosophical analysis of agent-based modelling: A new tool for theory development in nursing. *Journal of Advanced Nursing, 67*(4), 904–914.

Arslanian-Engoren, C., Hicks, F. D., Whall, A. L., & Algase, D. L. (2005). An ontological view of advanced practice nursing. *Research and Theory for Nursing Practice: An International Journal, 19*(4), 315–322.

Baird, D. (2004). *Thing knowledge: A philosophy of scientific instruments.* Berkeley: University of California Press.

Bluemel, K. (2004). *George Orwell and the radical eccentrics: Intermodernism in literary London.* New York, NY: Palgrave Macmillan.

Bohman, J. (2016). Critical theory. In E. N. Zalta (Ed.), *The Stanford encyclopedia of philosophy.* Retrieved from http://plato.stanford.edu/archives/fall2016/entries/critical-theory

Burns, J. (2014). The neomodernism approach: Professional development of baccalaureate level nurses–Influence of the metaparadigm of nursing on professional identity development among RN-BSN students. *Nursing Science Quarterly, 27*(1), 86–87.

Carter, B., & New, C. (Eds.). (2004). *Making realism work.* New York, NY: Routledge.

Cartwright, N. (1999). *The dappled world: A study of the boundaries of science.* Cambridge, England: University of Cambridge.

Clarke, B., James, C., & Kelly, J. (1996). Reflective practice: Reviewing the issues and refocusing the debate. *International Journal of Nursing Studies, 33*(2), 171–180.

Concise Routledge Encyclopedia of Philosophy. (2000). New York, NY: Routledge.

Conner, C. D. (2005). *A people's history of science: Miners, midwives, and low mechanics.* New York, NY: Nation Books.

Crotty, M. (1998). *The foundations of social research.* Thousand Oaks, CA: Sage.

Dant, T. (2003). *Critical social theory: Culture, society and critique.* Thousand Oaks, CA: Sage.

Darden, L. (2009). Discovering mechanisms in molecular biology: Finding and fixing incompleteness and incorrectness. In J. Meheus & T. Nickles (Eds.), *Models of discovery and creativity* (pp. 43–55). New York, NY: Springer.

Dickoff, J., & James, P. (1968). A theory of theories: A position paper. *Nursing Research, 17*(3), 197–203.

Diers, D. (2004). Clinical scholarship. In D. Diers (Ed.), *Speaking of nursing: Narratives of practice, research, policy and the profession* (pp. 79–89). Boston, MA: Jones & Bartlett. (Reprinted from Diers, D. (1995). Clinical scholarship. *Journal of Professional Nursing, 11*(1), 24–30.)

Doane, G. H., Browne, A. J., Reimer, J., MacLeod, M., & MacLellan, E. (2009). Enacting nursing obligations: Public health nurses' theorizing in practice. *Research and Theory for Nursing Practice: An International Journal, 23*(2), 88–106.

Doane, G. H., & Varcoe, C. (2005). Toward compassionate actions: Pragmatism and the inseparability of theory/practice. *Advances in Nursing Science, 28*(1), 81–90.

Ferris, T. (2010). *The science of liberty: Democracy*, reason, and the laws of nature. New York, NY: HarperCollins.

Gopnik, A. (2009). *Angels and ages: A short book about Darwin, Lincoln, and modern life.* New York, NY: Alfred A. Knopf.

Hanson, N. R. (1958). *Patterns of discovery: An inquiry into the conceptual foundations of science.* Cambridge, England: Cambridge University Press.

Hickman, L. A. (2007). *Pragmatism as post-postmodernism: Lessons from John Dewey.* New York, NY: Fordham University Press.

hooks, b. (1999). *Remembered rapture: Writer at work.* New York, NY: Henry Holt.

Johnson, R. (1993). Nurse practitioner-patient discourse: Uncovering the voice of nursing in primary care practice. *Scholarly Inquiry for Nursing Practice, 7,* 143–158.

Judd, D. M. (2009). *Questioning authority: Political resistance and the ethic of natural science.* New Brunswick, NJ: Transaction.

Kim, H. S. (1993). Practice theories in nursing and a science of nursing practice. *Scholarly Inquiry for Nursing Practice: An International Journal, 8*(2), 145–162.

Kim, H. S. (1999). Critical reflective inquiry for knowledge development in nursing practice. *Journal of Advanced Nursing, 29*(5), 1205–1212.

Kuhn, T. (1962). *The structure of scientific revolutions.* Chicago, IL: University of Chicago.

Latour, B. (1993). *We have never been modern* (C. Porter, Trans.). New York, NY: Harvester Wheatsheaf.

Latour, B., & Woolgar, S. (1986). *Laboratory life: The construction of scientific facts* (2nd ed.). Princeton, NJ: Princeton University Press.

Lewin, K. (1951). *Field theory in social science: Selected theoretical papers.* New York, NY: Harper & Row.

Liehr, P., & Smith, M. J. (2007). A neomodernist perspective for researching chronicity. *Archives in Psychiatric Nursing, 21*(6), 345–346.

Locsin, R. C. (2009). "Painting a clear picture": Technological knowing as a contemporary process of nursing. In R. C. Locsin & M. J. Purnell (Eds.), *A contemporary nursing process: The (un)bearable weight of knowing in nursing* (pp. 377–394). New York, NY: Springer Publishing.

Losse, J. (2004). *Theories of scientific progress.* New York, NY: Routledge.

Magee, B. (2001). *The story of philosophy* (2nd ed.). New York, NY: Dorling Kindersley.

McQueen, D. V. (2007). Critical issues in theory for health promotion. In D. V. McQueen & I. Kickbusch (Eds.), *Health and modernity: The role of theory in health promotion* (pp. 21–42). New York, NY: Springer.

Meheus, J., & Nickles, T. (Eds.). (2009). *Models of discovery and creativity.* New York, NY: Springer.

Montgomery, K. (2006). *How doctors think: Clinical judgment and the practice of medicine.* New York, NY: Oxford University Press.

Mouzelis, N. P. (2008). *Modern and postmodern social theorizing: Bridging the divide.* New York, NY: Cambridge University Press.

Neurath, O. (1983). Protocol statements. In R. S. Cohen & M. Neurath (Ed. & Trans.), *Philosophical papers: 1913–1946* (Vol. 16; pp. 91–99). Boston, MA: D. Reidel Publishing.

Oakley, A. (2000). *Experiments in knowing: Gender and method in the social sciences.* New York, NY: The New Press.

Peirce, C. S. (1934). *Charles Sanders Peirce: Collected papers* (Vol. 5), C. Hartshorne & P. Weiss (Eds.) (Vol. 7–8), A. W. Burks (Ed.). Cambridge, MA: Harvard University Press.

Peplau, H. E. (1952). *Interpersonal relations in nursing.* New York, NY: Putnam.

Peplau, H. E. (1987). Interpersonal constructs for nursing practice. *Nursing Education Today, 7*(95), 201–208.

Peplau, H. E. (1988). The art and science of nursing: Similarities, differences, and relations. *Nursing Science Quarterly, 1,* 8–15.

Peplau, H. E. (1992a). Interpersonal relations: A theoretical framework for application in nursing practice. *Nursing Science Quarterly, 5,* 13–18.

Peplau, H. E. (1992b). Perspectives on nursing knowledge (interview by T. Takahashi). *Nursing Science Quarterly, 5,* 86–91.

Petroski, H. (2010). *The essential engineer: Why science alone will not solve our global problems.* New York, NY: Alfred A. Knopf.

Pickering, A. (2005). *The mangle of practice: Time, agency and science.* Chicago, IL: University of Chicago Press.

Potvin, L., & Balbo, L. (2007). From a theory book to a theory group. In D. V. McQueen & I. Kickbusch (Eds.), *Health and modernity: The role of theory in health promotion* (pp. 6–11). New York, NY: Springer.

Råholm, M. (2010). Abductive reasoning and formation of scientific knowledge within nursing research. *Nursing Philosophy, 11,* 260–270.

Raymo, C. (2008). *When God is gone everything is holy: The making of a religious naturalist.* Notre Dame, IN: Sorin Books.

Reed, P. G. (1995). A treatise on nursing knowledge development for the 21st century: Beyond postmodernism. *Advances in Nursing Science, 17*(3), 70–84.

Reed, P. G. (1996). Transforming practice knowledge into nursing knowledge—A revisionist analysis of Peplau. *Image: Journal of Nursing Scholarship, 28*(1), 29–33.

Reed, P. G. (1997). Nursing: The ontology of the discipline. *Nursing Science Quarterly, 10*(2), 76–79.

Reed, P. G. (2006). Neomodernism and evidence based nursing: Implications for the production of nursing knowledge. *Nursing Outlook, 54*(1), 36–38.

Ritchie, D. E. (2010). *The fullness of knowing: Modernity and postmodernity from Defoe to Gadamer*. Waco, TX: Baylor University Press.

Smith, B. H. (2005). *Scandalous knowledge: Science, truth and the human*. Edinburgh, England: Edinburgh University Press.

Stepin, V. (2005). *Theoretical knowledge* (A. G. Georgiev & E. D. Rumiantseva, Trans.). Dordrecht, The Netherlands: Springer.

Tauber, A. I. (2009). *Science and the quest for meaning*. Waco, TX: Baylor University Press.

Thorne, S. (2005). Conceptualizing in nursing: What's the point? *Journal of Advanced Nursing, 5*(2), 107.

Van den Daele, W. (2004). Traditional knowledge in modern society. In N. Stehr (Ed.), *The governance of knowledge* (pp. 27–40). New Brunswick, NJ: Transaction.

Weissman, D. (2008). *Styles of thought: Interpretation, inquiry, and imagination*. New York, NY: SUNY Press.

Welt, S. R., & O'Toole, A. W. (1989). Hildegard E. Peplau: Observations in brief. *Archives of Psychiatric Nursing, 3*, 254–264.

Whall, A. L., & Hicks, F. D. (2002). The unrecognized paradigm shift in nursing: Implications, problems, and possibilities. *Nursing Outlook, 50*, 72–76.

Doctoral Nursing Roles in Knowledge Generation

Donna M. Velasquez, Donna Behler McArthur,
and Catherine Johnson

It has been nearly two decades since the Institute of Medicine (IOM, 2003) called for "a major overhaul" in the way health care professionals are educated to meet the challenge of improving health care in the 21st century. This challenge resulted in sweeping changes in health care education including the creation of a new doctoral degree for nursing, the doctor of nursing practice (DNP). The American Association of Colleges of Nursing (AACN) described the goal for DNP education as a "transformational change" for professional nurses who will practice at the most advanced level of nursing (AACN, 2006, p. 4). Although a master's degree remains entry level for nurse practitioners in all states, AACN and the National Organization of Nurse Practitioner Faculty (NONPF) have reaffirmed support of the DNP degree as the desired educational preparation for nurse practitioners (Melander, 2016). This support has contributed to the continued growth of DNP programs in the United States. In the past 5 years, the number of DNP programs has more than doubled to 273, with an additional 60 programs still planned (AACN, 2015).

When this chapter was first published in 2011, there was considerable concern within the discipline that despite the vision for practice at the highest level of practice outlined in *The Essentials of Doctoral Education for Advanced Nursing Practice* (*DNP Essentials*; AACN, 2006), there was not much difference in how advanced nursing practice had "been envisioned for the past several decades, except for the emphasis on the new knowledge outside of the discipline . . ." (Smith & McCarthy, 2010, p. 49).

More recently, knowledge from practice has gained some legitimacy and AACN has stated that "graduates of both research- and practice-focused doctoral programs are prepared to generate new knowledge" (AACN, 2015, p. 2).

This *knowledge from practice* concept is relatively new and there remain many questions about what DNP curriculum should encompass and the role of DNP prepared nurses (Staffileno, Murphy, & Carlson, 2017). Indeed, in a recent study by Dols, Hernández, and Miles (2017) ranking the importance of DNP project outcomes, some directors of DNP programs asked that "generation of new knowledge" be removed from the list as it was an outcome of research rather than DNP projects. Application of knowledge is at the philosophical core of practice doctorates such as the DNP, but there had been little discussion of the role of the DNP graduate in the generation of new knowledge from practice.

In this chapter, we present a conceptual model of a collaborative approach to delineating the practitioner–researcher and scientist–researcher roles in research and knowledge generation. We also present background and context surrounding our proposed model. There remains a significant gap in collaborations among PhD- and DNP-prepared nurses to conduct research and to translate knowledge to practice to improve patient outcomes. Our model delineates the distinct and shared contributions to the generation and application of knowledge by the DNP-prepared nurse as practitioner–theorist–researcher (PTR) and the PhD-prepared nurse as scientist–theorist–researcher (STR), which can serve to guide doctorally prepared nurse collaborations.

HISTORICAL PERSPECTIVES ON THE PRACTICE DOCTORATE

The concept of a practice doctorate is not new to nursing. Doctor of nursing science (DNS, DNSc) and nursing doctorate (ND) programs were introduced in the 1970s as clinical or practice-based degrees. However, with the exception of the ND program at Case Western Reserve University in Cleveland (which converted to a DNP in 2005), there is now little difference between most of these early practice doctorates and current research intensive PhD programs (Marion et al., 2003; Patzek, 2010). In an attempt to avoid a repeat of practice-based doctorates transitioning to research degrees, there has been an overemphasis on differentiating the two degrees while negating areas of overlap. This is especially apparent where there is an absence of content on philosophy, metatheory, and theory development and evaluation within DNP programs influenced by the AACN *Essentials of Doctoral Education for Advanced Nursing Practice* (AACN, 2006). This decreased emphasis places nursing at risk for losing a foundational understanding of the practice of nursing and becoming increasingly influenced by other disciplines (Whall, 2005). While the *Essentials* document calls for DNP graduates who are prepared to "develop and evaluate new practice approaches based on nursing theories . . ." (AACN, 2006, p. 9), reliance on nursing theory taught to students in their undergraduate or master's programs lacks sufficient depth to guide practice or for the generation of new knowledge and theory from practice.

DOCTORAL DEGREE NURSING AND KNOWLEDGE DEVELOPMENT

Historically, nursing followed the lead of the sciences, medicine, and other health care disciplines in placing highest value on the scientific empirical approach to creating new knowledge. In the 20th century, the philosophy of science that typically undergirded PhD programs emphasized research methods that produced context-free and replicable data. Because of this, many nurses conducted their research farther from the site of practice and from the providers of nursing care. However, scholars have increasingly questioned the relevance of these context-free data (Holloway & Wheeler, 2002; Rolfe, 1998) noting that expert practice involves making decisions within a particular context requiring knowledge of not only external evidence but also of "contextual and idiosyncratic" internal evidence (Avis & Freshwater, 2006, p. 223). The practice doctorate in nursing has helped stimulate movement away from strict adherence to traditional methods of research with new models of clinical knowledge generation and practice being envisioned.

EVIDENCE-BASED PRACTICE AND BEYOND

The nursing practice doctorate program leading to the DNP degree is designed to prepare experts in specialized advanced nursing practice. The DNP title does not designate a specialty; rather, DNP graduates are prepared for a variety of roles including leadership, administration, and advanced practice nursing (nurse practitioners, clinical nurse specialists, nurse anesthetists, and nurse midwives; AACN, 2006, p. 8). The focus is on practice that is innovative and evidence based, reflecting the application of credible research (AACN, 2006, p. 3).

EVIDENCE-BASED PRACTICE: HISTORY AND MODELS

Early models of research utilization predated the evidence-based practice (EBP) movement and should be appreciated as exemplars in narrowing the research–practice gap. Perhaps the best known project was the CURN (Conduct and Utilization of Research in Nursing) Project conducted by the Michigan Nurses' Association in the 1970s (Horsley, Crane, & Bingle, 1978). The goal was to increase the use of research in the practice of registered nurses within 20 hospitals. Findings from this project supported the relevance of using research in practice and forged the way for research utilization.

Sackett, Rosenberg, Gray, and Richardson (1996) described evidence-based medicine (EBM) as ancient in its origins, yet a relatively young discipline "whose positive impacts are just beginning to be validated" (p. 312). The term *EBM* was adopted by many disciplines including nursing but is now more commonly referred to as EBP in disciplines outside of medicine. Early criticism (and one that continues) included the equating of EBP with "cook-book" medicine. However, EBP goes beyond the mere adherence to published guidelines to combine thoughtful and systematic appraisal of multiple sources and levels of evidence. EBP is a problem-solving approach to clinical decision making within myriad health care arenas that integrates the best evidence from well-designed studies with the clinician's expertise, which includes internal evidence from patient assessments, patient data, and a patient's preferences and values (Melnyk, Fineout-Overholt, Gallagher-Ford, & Kaplan, 2012, p. 410). The goal of EBP is to promote effective nursing interventions, efficient care, and improved outcomes for patients, and to provide the best available evidence for clinical, administrative, and educational decision making (Newhouse, Dearholt, Poe, Pugh, & White, 2007, p. xiv).

Models of EBP have continued to emerge since the early 1980s including the Rosswurm-Larrabee Model of EBP (Rosswurm & Larrabee, 1999), the Iowa Model of Research in Practice (Titler et al., 2001), the Academic Center for Evidence-Based Practice (ACE) Star Model of Knowledge Transformation (Stevens, 2012), the Johns Hopkins Nursing EBP Model using the practice question, evidence, translation process (Newhouse et al., 2007), Advancing Research and Clinical Practice Through Close Collaboration (ARCC; Melnyk & Fineout-Overholt, 2002), Stetler Model (Stetler, 2001), and Promotion Action on Research Implementation in Health Services (PARIHS) framework (Rycroft-Malone, 2004). The PARIHS model has recently been refined and is now called the i-PARIHS framework. A core construct within the new framework is innovation, which is the focus of the implementation phase (Kitson & Harvey, 2016).

A comprehensive overview of EBP models and their practical applications for guiding change identified key EBP steps, features, and model classification (Schaffer, Sandau, & Diedrick, 2013). While purposes of the models vary, they all help the nurse organize thinking about how knowledge advances from basic discovery to application in practice whether at an organizational or individual level. Shared components of all models are determination of an identified need; data gathering; decision to accept, modify, or reject evidence; implementation; and evaluation. Desired outcomes are to maintain or improve patient health by reducing unnecessary variation in practice and improving quality and safety of care.

GOING BEYOND EXISTING MODELS

EBP is recognized as the cornerstone of clinical scholarship within nursing. Certainly most health care professionals would agree that care should be delivered based on information about what works. The challenge that remains is clarifying what evidence is and how this evidence is used in everyday decision making within the context of clinical practice. Furthermore, how theory and knowledge are generated from practice has not been well articulated.

One characteristic of a discipline is its distinct body of knowledge. Critics of EBP highlight the almost exclusive reliance of empirical knowledge while failing to consider other patterns of knowledge (NONPF, 2016; Porter, 2010). In contrast, DiCenso, Ciliska, and Guyatt (2005) posit that research use and research-based practice are subsets within the broader domain of evidence-based nursing (EBN). As such, Carper's (1978) ways of knowing in nursing (empirical, ethical, personal, and aesthetic) are included in the clinical decision-making process.

Further, knowledge is not developed in a linear manner. Theory leads to practice, but also practice leads to theory (Boyer, 1990). The outcomes of EBP within unique practice settings and contexts provide potential sources of new knowledge. Relying solely on models of EBP to guide nursing practice, with their emphasis on application of knowledge and their lack of processes for theory building and innovation, limits generation of knowledge. While research-based evidence is necessary for providing optimal care, it is not sufficient (Straus, Graham, & Mazmanian, 2006). Evidence is the foundation of practice; however, new and innovative delivery models are needed to generate new knowledge from practice (Porter-O'Grady & Malloch, 2017).

The AACN Task Force on the Implementation of the DNP (AACN, 2015) describes the practice-focused graduate as being prepared to generate new knowledge through the innovation of practice change, the translation of evidence, and the implementation of quality improvement processes in specific practice settings, systems, or with specific populations to improve health or health outcomes (p. 2). As clinical scholars, DNP-prepared advanced practice nurses use multiple sources of nursing knowledge to advance nursing practice and policy (NONPF, 2016).

A CONCEPTUAL MODEL OF DOCTORAL NURSING KNOWLEDGE GENERATION

To make way for practice-based knowledge generation, a new model for conceptualizing the relationship between nursing research and nursing practice is needed. New models for discipline-based research and practice have emerged in other health care disciplines and are designed to address the educational needs of expert practitioners as well as recognition of the changing research needs important to the discipline (Ragland, 2006; Stephan, 2006).

While tacit knowledge has long been accepted as legitimately created through practice, the significance of practice experiences in developing explicit new scientific knowledge has not been adequately recognized or promoted. Practice-based methods of nursing knowledge development require systematic observation, appropriate methodologies, and synthesis of evidence not unlike that required to develop knowledge in academic research settings. However, while basic processes of science are valued and shared by DNP and PhD nurses, there are important differences in the types of questions and use of methods suitable to complex practice environments. To help advance the idea that practitioners can and should do research, we have proposed a model that clarifies some of the distinctions and similarities between DNP- and PhD-prepared nurses, with particular focus on their roles in development of nursing knowledge. Within the model, there is an emphasis on collaboration between DNP- and PhD-prepared nurses and the resulting innovation.

ROLES IN PRACTICE AND RESEARCH

Jarvis (2000) was one of the first to claim that the "practitioner–researcher" model was critical for nursing given the increased emphasis on efficiencies of nursing practice and the widespread belief that a gap exists between nursing theory and nursing practice. Freshwater (2003) distinguished between the *practitioner–researcher* and the *scientist–researcher*. The scientist–researcher focuses on the development of explanatory, predictive theories to arrive at general statements about large areas of reality. The goal of the practitioner–researcher is problem solving and producing more specific statements about local and contingent situations (Freshwater, 2003, p. 4). We extended these ideas about doctoral nursing roles in our conceptual model to envision how all doctoral nurses may contribute to theory-based knowledge.

In our model, the domain of the DNP-prepared nurse is identified by the term *PTR* while the domain of the PhD-prepared nurse is identified in the model as *STR* (Figure 3.1). The addition of *theorist* in each domain was done to acknowledge that all

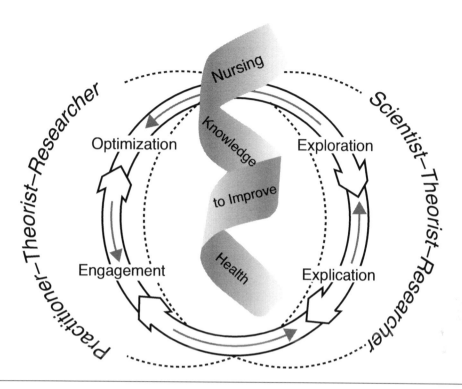

FIGURE 3.1 Conceptual model of doctoral nursing roles in knowledge generation.

doctorally prepared nurses, whether predominantly practitioners or academicians, make contributions to nursing theory. This idea of the practitioner as theorist is not new. As Rosemary Ellis (1969) explained, if nurses are to move beyond "the personal accumulation of wisdom from patient to patient" (p. 1438), practitioners must be willing to become scholars to develop and test theories derived from practice. Building on this, Reed (2008) advanced the notion of the "practitioner as theorist" introducing new perspectives for developing theory from practice. It is through practice that the relevance of nursing theories is determined. Nurses are educated into understanding that they can apply or adapt existing theories, as well as develop new theories from systematic observations in practice settings to be applied, tested, and ultimately transformed into nursing knowledge (Reed, 2008).

The two outer circles in the model (depicted by dotted lines) represent the two domains, STR and PTR, which comprise core roles for knowledge generation. A key dynamic represented by the intersecting circles is the permeability of boundaries between the STR and PTR to not only reduce role constraints but also facilitate knowledge flow between academic and practitioner communities with the creation of partnerships and collaborations. While Baumbusch et al. (2008) and many others have emphasized the reciprocity and exchange between producers and users of knowledge, we propose that being solely a producer or a user of knowledge is untenable for doctoral nurses; the STR and PTR alike must participate in knowledge production. PTRs are uniquely positioned to observe firsthand patient responses to health care processes and interventions and, therefore, are in a key position to not only apply but also generate new knowledge and theories. Rather than perpetuate the role of the handmaiden, whether to the theory-based knowledge of the physician or to the knowledge produced by the PhD-prepared nurse, the model depicts the PTR as an equal partner in knowledge and theory development to improve human health. Thus, the addition of the PTR role for DNP graduates broadens nursing's resources for knowledge development through distinct and shared contributions of both doctoral nurse roles.

SYNTHESIZING EXISTING MODELS OF PRACTICE KNOWLEDGE DEVELOPMENT

We developed our conceptual model by synthesizing ideas from the literature as well as through reflection on our own practices. We drew some ideas from two existing models of knowledge development in practice: the ACE Star Model (Stevens, 2004) and translational research models (Woolf, 2006).

The ACE Star Model of Knowledge Transformation (Stevens, 2012) depicts knowledge as evidence from research combined with extant knowledge from other sources and integrated into practice. The stages of knowledge development include knowledge discovery, evidence summary, translation, integration, and evaluation. The emphasis is on transforming large amounts of basic knowledge into a form useful for everyday clinical decision making to improve patient outcomes (Stevens, 2012; Stevens & Staley, 2006).

Several translational research models have been published. For many, the meaning of translational research is limited to the translation of basic science into drugs, devices, and new medical treatments (from bench to bedside; Woolf, 2006). However, just as EBP is applied widely across disciplines and professions, translational science has application beyond the discipline of medicine. Translational research is more broadly defined as the "overarching principle of judicious application of synthesized knowledge to improve health outcomes for individuals and the health care system" (Graham & Tetroe, 2007; Straus et al., 2006; Vincent, Johnson, Velasquez, & Rigney, 2010).

While models of translational research vary in number of steps or stages, all begin with basic or discovery research referred to as T1. Discovery (T1) research is the focus and recipient of the majority of federal funding and is performed by clinical scientists with mastery of basic sciences (Woolf, 2006). T2 (and additional phases beyond T1 depending on the particular translational model) are concerned with the implementation, evaluation, and dissemination of knowledge to influence everyday decision making by the practitioner. "T2 struggles more with human behavior and organizational inertia, infrastructure and resource constraints, and the messiness of proving effectiveness" (Woolf, 2006, p. 212) within complex environments that cannot be neatly controlled.

The strength of EBP and translational models in explicating knowledge-development approaches among DNP- and PhD-prepared nurses is that they clearly describe processes of advancing knowledge from research to practice. However, the focus in these models is on the application of knowledge handed down from the basic sciences while failing to capture the dynamic process of knowledge and theory generated from practice (Nonaka, Toyama, & Konna, 2000).

PHASES OF KNOWLEDGE DEVELOPMENT IN PRACTICE

Within our model, four phases are depicted: *exploration, explication, engagement,* and *optimization.* Theory and knowledge development are recognized as occurring across all phases—not only in the exploration and explication phases but continuing into practice as characterized by the phases of engagement and optimization.

Exploration represents the phase of knowledge development that has traditionally been referred to as the process of knowledge discovery (Boyer, 1990). Theory is generated to explain some phenomena using conventional research methods to systematically obtain quantitative and qualitative data. Typically, in the Western science paradigm, PhD scholars in academic settings have been recognized as the primary knowledge producers. However, this paradigm is shifting and knowledge production is increasingly viewed as distributed throughout society (Bartunek, Trullen, Bonet, & Sauquet, 2003). Within our conceptual model, this phase represents a primary, but not exclusive, domain of the PhD-prepared nurse.

Explication includes testing a proposed theory or interventions under ideal circumstances and where internal validity is a key concern. Explication is somewhat analogous to theory evaluation in which strengths and weaknesses are uncovered through a process of testing and examining outcomes in reality although the "reality" in this stage is still closely controlled and effects of context are minimized to increase internal validity. The methods of knowledge development associated with this phase typically have been emphasized more in PhD than in DNP curricula. However, nursing research often stagnates at this phase as few academic researchers have the opportunity to fully integrate knowledge and theory into sustainable practice.

Engagement refers to the meshing and integration of knowledge into practice. For this phase we extended the notion of integration presented in the ACE Star Model. Our use of the term goes beyond the integration of knowledge developed through basic research. Engagement in our model describes a dynamic process that implies the commitment of participants to implementation, evaluation, and dissemination of knowledge as it is applied in practice and to the generation of new knowledge from practice. This process requires understanding nursing theory, systems, and methods suitable for complex practice environments. Knowledge and theory are not only applied, but are also generated in this phase through action and interaction among individuals and organizations (Nonaka et al., 2000). Knowledge of innovation theories, knowledge translation, program evaluation, and quality improvement methodologies are central to this phase. DNP curricula that emphasize these areas uniquely prepare DNP graduates to use these methods to lead knowledge development.

Optimization is the phase in which knowledge and theory generation is viewed as dynamic and ongoing, continuously inspiring new questions and innovations. Optimization is the process of maximizing the effectiveness of an intervention in the practice setting. Interventions are revised and refined until they are optimal for a specific context, culture, and population. This is an ongoing process requiring a "flexible, responsive, and subjective approach" to knowledge production (Rolfe & Davies, 2009, p. 1271). Through the process of revision and refinement, new questions or problems may stimulate exploration. However, not all problems will require a return to the exploration phase; instead, knowledge generated in this phase may lead to changes in health policy, or other changes at the organizational, unit, or individual levels—all of which capitalize on DNP graduate role preparation.

SUMMARIZING THE STRUCTURAL ELEMENTS OF THE CONCEPTUAL MODEL

Within our model, a central circle depicts the dynamic process of nursing knowledge development across the four phases: *exploration, explication, engagement,* and *optimization.* The process is not necessarily linear as indicated by forward and backward arrows. The forward arrows suggest the traditional notion of knowledge as it is generated and transformed from basic discovery through application and evaluation. However, poor or unexpected outcomes may necessitate a return to the previous phase, indicated by backward arrows. The area marked by the intersection of the two circles represents knowledge generated through the action and interaction of various methodologies, collaborations, and disciplinary knowledge foundational to both roles of doctorally prepared nurses.

Although the inner circle depicts an orderly movement of knowledge from one phase to the next, a central spiral is used to characterize the synergy and "messiness" (nonlinearity) that occurs among the stages and across roles. While exploration and explication are primarily viewed as domains of the STR and engagement and optimization the domains of the PTR, boundaries are permeable and flexible as indicated by the dotted lines of the two outer circles. Both nursing roles may engage in any of the methods that constitute the phases. While the flexibility and permeability of roles add complexity to our concept of knowledge generation, it is meant to indicate the differences between PhD and DNP educational programs while recognizing that learning is not bounded to formal degree programs. That is, the PhD- and DNP-prepared nurses may extend their research practices beyond those traditional methods learned in their programs, to learn to use the methods of the *other* knowledge-development domain.

IMPLICATIONS FOR CURRICULUM: PRACTICE-BASED KNOWLEDGE DEVELOPMENT

This proposed model has curricular implications for particular areas of knowledge and skills needed by the PTR beyond those typically taught across DNP programs today. *The Essentials of Doctoral Education for Advanced Nursing Practice* (AACN, 2006) emphasizes the scholarly role of the DNP graduate through integration and application of knowledge. However, we maintain that for health care to be transformed, knowledge generated through practice must continue to be legitimized and valorized. The doctoral nursing curriculum is one important place to initiate this movement. Missing from the *DNP Essentials*, the foundation for DNP programs is the intensive and extensive emphasis on disciplinary knowledge through the study of theory and practice models (Smith & McCarthy, 2010).

Knowledge about the philosophy and theories of nursing science help create a common language necessary for communication within the discipline. Nursing has learned the language of medicine and other disciplines to enable interdisciplinary collaboration, but there remains a communication gap *within* nursing contributing to the theory–practice gap which inhibits collaboration between DNP- and PhD-prepared nurses. An understanding of nursing theory and research related to knowledge-development practices may better enable nurses to translate knowledge not only from other disciplines but from nursing science as well. There is a need to develop theory-building strategies that "have fit and relevance in practice" (Reed, 2008, p. 317), which are enhanced by the combined perspectives of the STR and PTR nurses.

Our conceptual model of knowledge and theory generation provides a model for developing curricula to teach the content and skills needed to develop new knowledge through research and practice while continuing to recognize knowledge and theory from other disciplines. Content emphasizing nursing theory, clinical practice, nursing research and evaluation methods, critical reflection, decision making, and collaboration will prepare DNP graduates to more fully assume their role as PTR.

ENVISIONING THE FUTURE OF KNOWLEDGE DEVELOPMENT AND NURSING PRACTICE

The nature of clinical practice is changing rapidly while the interactions between practitioners and clients maintain their uniqueness. Nevertheless, it is within this practice environment that practitioners may creatively synthesize all evidence available to them to construct an innovative approach to the care of individuals and patient populations. It is also within this environment that relevant pragmatic clinical research is both needed and possible. Purposeful utilization and evaluation of evidence obtained in the clinical setting by the PTR can legitimize the evidence and expand the knowledge base beyond local practice.

The goal of the practice doctorate in nursing is to create the highest level of practitioner (AACN, 2006). However, this may entail more attention to developing the tools of scholarship and knowledge development than originally conceived. "A doctorally prepared [nursing] graduate is expected to both utilize and develop knowledge" (Dracup, Cronenwett, Meleis, & Benner, 2005, p. 179), whether the nurse is prepared with a DNP, PhD, or other nursing doctoral degree. Clinical scholarship practice by the DNP will not be achieved by merely supplementing current master's level curriculums with a few additional courses. Instead, a curricula that incorporates theory, research, and practice methodologies suited to complex practice environments and, at the same time, supports development of excellent clinicians are needed to move EBP from a "cook-book" approach to a conscientious, caring, and scientific process to improve health care.

Our conceptual model proposes a collaborative approach to knowledge development by delineating and interconnecting PTR and STR roles. Both are needed to best serve nursing's goal of practicing at the highest level to improve health. Academic DNP and PhD programs have an opportunity to build models of collaboration and shared research that not only demonstrate a breadth of knowledge generation strategies but also encourage and guide collaboration among nursing experts. Our conceptual model represents one way to move forward in thinking about the roles of all doctorally prepared nurses in knowledge development for the discipline of nursing.

SUMMARY POINTS

1. The practitioner–researcher and the scientist–researcher both have roles in research and knowledge generation from and for practice.

2. Relying solely on EBP models to guide nursing practice, with their emphasis on application of knowledge and their lack of attention to generation of knowledge, is insufficient for providing optimal care.

3. The authors' conceptual model delineates the distinct and shared contributions to the generation and application of knowledge by the DNP-prepared nurse as PTR and the PhD-prepared nurse as STR.

4. Purposeful utilization and evaluation of evidence obtained in the clinical setting by the PTR can legitimize the evidence and expand the knowledge base beyond local practice.

QUESTIONS FOR REFLECTION

1. In looking at the conceptual model and thinking about your practice experiences,

    • What are some of the challenges that you might face engaging in the roles to build knowledge?

    • What are problems or areas of interest that you would like to see studied in your practice setting?

2. The chapter outlined four phases in knowledge generation, which can be shared by DNP and PhD nurses. What type of questions and methods are suitable for the complex practice environment based on your experience or readings?

3. A collaborative approach to research in delineating the practitioner–researcher and scientist–researcher roles has been proposed in this chapter. How might you use the model in your own practice to move nursing knowledge forward in a new way?

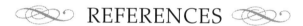 REFERENCES

American Association of Colleges of Nursing. (2006). *The essentials of doctoral education for advanced nursing practice.* Washington, DC: Author.

American Association of Colleges of Nursing. (2015). *The doctor of nursing practice: Current issues and clarifying recommendations.* Washington, DC: Author.

Avis, M., & Freshwater, D. (2006). Evidence for practice, epistemology, and critical reflection. *Nursing Philosophy, 7,* 216–224.

Bartunek, J., Trullen, J., Bonet, E., & Sauquet, A. (2003). Sharing and expanding academic and practitioner knowledge in health care. *Journal of Health Services Research & Policy, 8*(S2), 62–68.

Baumbusch, J. L., Kirkham, S. R., Khan, K. B., McDonald, H., Semeniuk, P., Tan, E., & Anderson, J. M. (2008). Pursuing common agendas: A collaborative model for knowledge translation between research and practice in clinical settings. *Research in Nursing & Health, 31,* 130–140.

Boyer, E. (1990). *Scholarship reconsidered: Priorities for the American professoriate.* Princeton, NJ: Carnegie Foundation for the Advancement of Teaching.

Carper, B. A. (1978). Fundamental patterns of knowing in nursing. *Advances in Nursing Science, 1*(1), 13–23.

DiCenso, A., Ciliska, D., & Guyatt, G. (2005). Introduction to evidence-based nursing. In A. DiCenso, G. Guyatt, & D. Ciliska (Eds.), *Evidence-based nursing: A guide to clinical practice* (pp. 3–19). St. Louis, MO: Elsevier Mosby.

Dols, J. D., Hernández, C., & Miles, H. (2017). The DNP project: Quandaries for nursing scholars. *Nursing Outlook, 65*(1), 84–93.

Dracup, K., Cronenwett, L., Meleis, A. I., & Benner, P. E. (2005). Reflections on the doctorate of nursing practice. *Nursing Outlook, 3*, 177–182.

Ellis, R. (1969). Practitioner as theorist. *American Journal of Nursing, 69*, 1434–1438.

Freshwater, D. (2003). Understanding and implementing clinical nursing research. *Proceedings of the 2003 ICN Biennial Conference, Switzerland*. Retrieved from http://citeseerx.ist.psu.edu/viewdoc/summary?doi=10.1.1.117.3351

Graham, I. D., & Tetroe, J. (2007). Whither knowledge translation. *Nursing Research, 56*(4S), S86–S88.

Holloway, I., & Wheeler, S. (2002). *Qualitative research in nursing*. Oxford, United Kingdom: Blackwell Science.

Horsley, J. A., Crane, J., & Bingle, J. (1978). Research utilization as an organizational process. *Journal of Nursing Administration, 8*(7), 4–6.

Institute of Medicine. (2003). *Health professions education: A bridge to quality*. Washington, DC: National Academies Press.

Jarvis, P. (2000). The practitioner-researcher in nursing. *Nurse Education Today, 20*, 30–35.

Kitson, A. L., & Harvey, G. (2016). Methods to succeed in effective knowledge translation to clinical practice. *Journal of Nursing Scholarship, 48*(3), 294–302.

Marion, L., Viens, D., O'Sullivan, A. L., Crabtree, K., Fontana, S., & Price, M. M. (2003). The practice doctorate in nursing: Future or fringe? *Topics in Advanced Practice Nursing eJournal*. Retrieved from http://www.medscape.com/viewarticle/453247

Melander, S. D. (2016). The president's message. Retrieved from http://www.nonpf.org/?page=31

Melnyk, B. M., & Fineout-Overholt, E. (2002). Rochester ARCC: Putting research into practice. *Reflections on Nursing Leadership, Sigma Theta Tau International, Honor Society of Nursing, 28*(2), 22–25.

Melnyk, B. M., Fineout-Overholt, E., Gallagher-Ford, L., & Kaplan, L. (2012). The state of evidence-based practice in US nurses. *The Journal of Nursing Administration, 42*(9), 410–417.

National Organization of Nurse Practitioner Faculty. (2016). White paper: The doctor of nursing practice nurse practitioner clinical scholar. Retrieved from http://c.ymcdn.com/sites/www.nonpf.org/resource/resmgr/docs/ClinicalScholarFINAL2016.pdf.

Newhouse, R., Dearholt, S., Poe, S., Pugh, L., & White, K. (2007). *Johns Hopkins nursing evidence-based practice—Model and guidelines*. Indianapolis, IN: Sigma Theta Tau.

Nonaka, I., Toyama, R., & Konna, N. (2000). SECI, Ba and leadership: A unified model of dynamic knowledge creation. *Long Range Planning, 33*, 5–34.

Patzek, M. J. (2010). Understanding the DNP degree. *American Nurse Today, 5*(5), 49–50.

Porter, S. (2010). Fundamental patterns of knowing in nursing: The challenge of evidence-based practice. *Advances in Nursing Science, 33*(1), 3–14.

Porter-O'Grady, T., & Malloch, K. (2017). Evidence-based practice and the innovation paradigm: A model for the continuum of practice excellence. In S. Davidson, D. Weberg, T. Porter-O'Grady, & K. Malloch (Eds.), *Leadership for evidence-based innovation in nursing and health professions* (pp. 3–41). Burlington, MA: Jones & Bartlett.

Ragland, B. (2006). Positioning the practitioner-researcher. *Action Research, 4*(2), 165–182.

Reed, P. G. (2008). Practitioner as theorist: A reprise. *Nursing Science Quarterly, 21*(4), 315–321.

Rolfe, G. (1998). The theory-practice gap in nursing: From research-based practice to practice-based research. *Journal of Advanced Nursing, 28*(3), 672–679.

Rolfe, G., & Davies, R. (2009). Second generation professional doctorates in nursing. *International Journal of Nursing Studies, 46*, 1265–1273.

Rosswurm, M. A., & Larrabee, J. H. (1999). A model for change to evidence-based practice. *Image: Journal of Nursing Scholarship, 31*(4), 317–322.

Rycroft-Malone. (2004). The PARIHS framework—A framework for guiding the implementation of evidence-based practice. *Journal of Nursing Care Quality, 19*(4), 297–304.

Sackett, D., Rosenberg, W., Gray, J., & Richardson, W. (1996). Evidence based medicine: What it is and what it is not. *British Medical Journal, 312*, 71–72.

Schaffer, M. A., Sandau, K. E., & Diedrick, L. (2013). Evidence-based practice models for organizational change: Overview and practical applications. *Journal of Advanced Nursing, 69*(5), 1197–1209.

Smith, M., & McCarthy, M. P. (2010). Disciplinary knowledge in nursing education: Going beyond the blueprints. *Nursing Outlook, 58*, 44–51.

Staffileno, B. A., Murphy, M. P., & Carlson, E. (2017). Determinants for effective collaboration among DNP- and PhD-prepared faculty. *Nursing Outlook, 65*(1), 94–102.

Stephan, W. (2006). Bridging the researcher-practitioner divide in intergroup relations. *Journal of Social Issues, 62*(63), 597–605.

Stetler, C. (2001). Updating the Stetler model of research utilization to facilitate evidence-based practice. *Nursing Outlook, 49*, 272–278.

Stevens, K. R. (2012). *The Star Model of Knowledge Transformation*. Retrieved from http://nursing.uthscsa.edu/onrs/starmodel/star-model.asp

Stevens, K. R., & Staley, J. M. (2006). The Quality Chasm reports, evidence-based practice, and nursing's response to improve healthcare. *Nursing Outlook, 54*, 94–101.

Straus, S. E., Graham, I. D., & Mazmanian, P. E. (2006). Knowledge translation: Resolving the confusion. *The Journal of Continuing Education in the Health Professions, 26*(1), 3–4.

Titler, M. G., Kleiber, C., Steelman, V., Rakel, B., Budreau, G., Everett, L. O., . . . Goode, C. J. (2001). The Iowa model of evidence-based practice to promote quality care. *Critical Care Nursing Clinics of North America, 13*(4), 497–509.

Vincent, D., Johnson, C., Velasquez, D., & Rigney, T. (2010). DNP as "practitioner-researcher": Closing the gap between research and practice. *The American Journal for Nurse Practitioners, 14*(11/12), 24–28.

Whall, A. L. (2005). "Lest we forget": An issue concerning the doctorate of nursing practice (DNP). *Nursing Outlook, 53*, 1.

Woolf, S. H. (2006). The meaning of translational research and why it matters. *Journal of the American Medical Association, 299*(2), 211–213.

Practitioner-Centered Research: Nursing Praxis and the Science of the Unique

| Gary Rolfe |

It is perhaps disingenuous of me to begin a chapter on practitioner research in nursing practice with this particular quote from T. S. Eliot, since he was bemoaning the very "endless cycle of idea and action, endless invention, endless experiment" (Eliot, 1934/1940) that I intend to advocate. When Eliot used the word *wisdom*, he was referring to the outcome of a process of silent internal contemplation that he identified as prayer, but which, in the secular world of nursing practice, we might describe as reflection-on-action (Schön, 1983), the thoughtful contemplation of prior practice. However, this chapter is concerned with another form of wisdom that arises from another form of reflection; that is, with the clinical wisdom or wise action that results from Schön's (1983) reflection-*in*-action or on-the-spot experimenting.

I intend to use Eliot's ascending hierarchy of information, knowledge, and wisdom as a framework for my critique of the current paradigm of nursing research and evidence-based practice (EBP) and my subsequent exploration of nursing praxis, the integration of research and practice in the clinical setting. I suggest in particular that the move toward EBP as the underpinning rationale for clinical nursing has led to an abandonment of the search for wisdom, and even for knowledge and theory, in favor of the accumulation of information about the comparative effectiveness and efficiency of different nursing interventions.

Eliot was right to point out that the descent from wisdom to information entails a loss. However, there is a real danger for nursing that the loss is not recognized and that practitioners act in the mistaken belief that wise actions can be reconstituted from information that has had all of the rich, contextual personal knowledge stripped from it. As educationalist Lawrence Stenhouse (1978) warned,

> Without understanding why one course of action is better than another, we could prove by statistical treatment that it is. The vision is an enticing one: it suggests that we may make wise judgments without understanding what we are doing. (p. 28)

The purpose of this chapter is to argue that the social and medical research paradigms adopted by the academic discipline of nursing are no longer fit for purpose in the 21st century and to propose that we consider in their place a science of the unique person underpinned by praxis, the coming together of research and practice in a single, seamless act.

ACADEMIC NURSING AND THE RISE OF NURSING THEORY

As with many emerging professions, the advent of modern nursing in the mid-19th century was preceded by many years before its acceptance as a full academic discipline. The date and manner of the entry of nursing into the academy is open to dispute but might for convenience be taken as 1923 when Yale opened the first independent university-based school for the education of nurses. However, if we measure the maturity of an academic discipline by the widespread award of master's and doctoral degrees, then the discipline of nursing only came of age in the 1970s in the United States (Kalisch & Kalisch, 2004) and even later in other parts of the world.

Prior to its entry into the academy, the theoretical underpinning of the practice of nursing consisted predominantly of Nightingale's twin pillars of public health and compassionate caring (Nightingale, 1860). However, many of the early master's programs in nursing admitted graduates in disciplines other than nursing, culminating in a generation of nurse academics who brought with them a range of theories and methods from other disciplines, mostly in the social sciences. This in turn led to a broadening out of theoretical perspectives and a particular emphasis on social science research paradigms as the primary means of conceptualizing and generating nursing knowledge. More recently, the EBP movement has heralded a move away from grand and middle-range theory generation and testing in nursing toward a more pragmatic and eclectic approach in which nursing practice is shaped and directed predominantly according to the findings of quantitative evaluation studies and randomized trials.

The term *nursing research* is therefore nowadays applied to two separate and in many ways distinct fields of scholarly activity. On one hand, many nurse researchers continue to employ the methods and methodologies of the social sciences, particularly from sociology and anthropology, to develop, test, and modify nursing theory. On the other hand, a small but growing group of researchers are using the experimental and quasi-experimental methodologies derived from medicine and (as we shall see) agriculture to test the effectiveness and efficacy of specific nursing interventions in clinical trials. These two groups of nurse researchers often come into conflict, with the social scientists claiming that the experimentalists have no regard for theory and the traditions of nursing, and the experimentalists claiming that the social scientists are advocating practice that is not based on robust and rigorous scientific evidence.

While the methods and methodologies of each camp have their uses and have undoubtedly made valuable contributions to the practice of nursing, I suggest in this chapter that neither of them is sufficiently grounded in nursing practice to make the claim to be fully "nursing research." In particular, I argue that whereas the methods and methodologies of social research and clinical trials have evolved to meet the needs of the social sciences and medicine, respectively, nursing practice has a very different agenda and focus from either of these disciplines and requires a very different approach to the generation and application of knowledge. Indeed, I suggest that a discipline such as nursing, whose focus and goals revolve around practice, requires a different understanding not only of how knowledge should be generated but also of what knowledge *is*. This in turn implies a radical reconceptualization of what it means to be an academic discipline (and, on a personal level, what it means to be an academic) in a practice-based profession. This challenge is set out clearly by Donald Schön (1983) in his investigation into the demands of "professional education," that is, education for practice:

> We are in need of inquiry into an epistemology of practice. What is the kind of knowing in which competent practitioners engage? How is professional knowing like and unlike the kinds of knowledge presented in academic textbooks, scientific papers, and learned journals? In what sense, if any, is there intellectual rigor in professional practice? (p. viii)

This chapter attempts to address some of Schön's (1983) questions and outlines a new epistemology of nursing that pays attention, in Schön's words, to the kind of knowing in which competent practitioners engage. This task includes not only an examination of what practitioners need to know but also of the ways in which that knowledge is constructed and what, if anything, should count as intellectual rigor in a discipline for which the focus of inquiry is ultimately the development of practice rather than theory. In short, this chapter proposes and explores the argument that most of the research methods and methodologies currently considered to be central to the discipline of nursing are, in fact, *fundamentally* unsuitable and ill-equipped to generate the kinds of knowledge that nurses require for practice in the 21st century.

NURSING AND THE SOCIAL SCIENCES

A brief scan through the contents pages of any of the major nursing research textbooks from the past 30 years or so will confirm that nursing research has become intimately associated with the methodologies and methods of the social sciences, particularly with sociology and anthropology. This has been due in part to the generally accepted definition of nursing as a social activity and in part to a significant number of prominent and influential nurse academics having had a prior grounding in various social science disciplines and their respective research methods and methodologies. I therefore begin with a discussion of the aims of social research and an exploration of how they differ from the requirements of nursing practice.

It is widely accepted by social scientists that the primary and perhaps sole purpose of social research is to generate, test, and inform social knowledge and theory, and it has usually been considered sufficient merely to change the word *social* to *nursing* to produce a paradigm for nursing research. I suggest that this uncritical embracing of the methodologies of social research into nursing is problematic in a number of ways. First, it immediately sets out the expectation that nursing and the social sciences should share similar aims, methods, and epistemologies and, indeed, that nursing *is* a social science. Second, it assumes that the primary function and purpose of nursing research should be to produce nursing knowledge. Third, it implies that research can only inform practice through the medium of knowledge and theory and thus locates practice at least one degree removed from research. Fourth, and following on from this assumption, it suggests that the kinds of knowledge generated by the social science research methods and methodologies can be applied in a more or less direct and unproblematic way to nursing practice.

The relationship outlined previously between research on one hand and knowledge and theory on the other has been accepted more or less uncritically in nursing and has subsequently become so entrenched as to be almost axiomatic. To suggest that the purpose of nursing research might be *something other* than to produce or test nursing knowledge and (to a lesser extent) nursing theory is generally considered misguided at best and heretical at worst. Thus, Polit and Beck (2004) defined nursing research as "systematic inquiry designed to develop *knowledge* about issues of importance to the nursing profession" and clinical nursing research as "designed to generate *knowledge* to guide nursing practice and to improve the health and quality of life of nurses' clients" (p. 3, emphasis added). In the most recent edition of this text, "knowledge" has been replaced by "trustworthy evidence" (Polit & Beck, 2017), suggesting a further shift down T. S. Eliot's hierarchy away from wisdom and knowledge, toward information. The essence of these definitions is repeated throughout the literature, and it is widely accepted that the purpose of nursing research is predominantly to generate knowledge (and, more recently, evidence) that can be employed by nurses to enhance their practice.

Implicit in this conception of nursing research is a one-way hierarchical relationship in which research leads to improved knowledge and knowledge leads to improved practice. This in turn implies a similar one-way hierarchical relationship between researchers and practitioners, where nurses are expected to base their practice primarily on the work of academics who are often no longer (or, indeed, may never have been) clinically active. As Greenwood (1966) pointed out nearly half a century ago:

> In the evolution of every profession there emerges the researcher-theoretician whose role is that of scientific investigation and theoretical systematization. In technological professions, a division of labor thereby evolves between the theory-oriented and the practice-oriented person. (p. 12)

Priyjmachuk (1996) added that, in the discipline of nursing, "it is the theories of the pure scientists that dictate the actions of those in practice," and "though a relationship between theory and practice appears to exist, it seems somewhat unidirectional in nature" (p. 680). Schön (1983) referred to this unidirectional flow of knowledge from research to practice in the professions as technical rationality. While such a hierarchical relationship between research and practice and between researchers and practitioners might be appropriate in the social science disciplines, it is far less straightforward when the social science research methodologies are applied to practice disciplines such as nursing, for which they were never originally intended.

The main difficulty with applying the findings from social research methodologies to the practice of nursing becomes immediately apparent when we consider the purpose for which social research was originally developed. Sociology has been defined in simple terms as "the scientific study of human life, social groups, whole societies and the human world" (Giddens & Sutton, 2013, p. 43).

The original purpose of social research was to understand and predict the *collective behavior* of social groups and societies to inform practical and policy decisions about social institutions and relationships. Even in social science disciplines such as anthropology, where the focus is often on small and sometimes idiosyncratic groups and organizations, the aim is usually to produce an objective and scientific account that allows us to make inferences to human behavior *in general*. Thus

> The culture can be turned into an object available for study . . . [and] it is possible to construct an account of the culture under investigation that both understands it from within and captures it as external to, and independent of, the researcher; in other words, as a natural phenomenon. (Hammersley & Atkinson, 2007, p. 9)

The implications of this description are first that anthropology can be safely regarded as an objective science and second that it is akin to the natural sciences insofar as culture is presented as a widespread and naturally occurring phenomenon. These twin assumptions allowed the founding mothers and fathers of cultural anthropology to make the claim that it enabled "advanced" societies to understand the history of their own social development by studying cultures that are operating at a supposedly more "primitive" level, in much the same way that paleontologists can trace biological development by studying primitive organisms.

Even the more ideographic social research methodologies such as phenomenology can be seen to be underpinned by realist and/or positivist assumptions about essence and generalizability. Thus

> Phenomenological researchers ask: What is the *essence* of this phenomenon as experienced by these people and what does it *mean*? Phenomenologists assume there is an essence—an essential invariant structure—that can be understood, in much the same way that ethnographers assume that cultures exist. Phenomenologists investigate subjective phenomena in the belief that critical *truths about reality* are grounded in people's lived experiences. (Polit & Beck, 2006, p. 219, emphasis added)

The stated purpose of phenomenology, at least as it is presented here, is to uncover truths about reality through a process of "bracket[ing] out the world and any presuppositions in an effort to confront the data in pure form" (Polit & Beck, 2006, p. 220). Although phenomenologists typically work with small samples, the aim is to make universal statements about essential truths based on common categories of "lived experiences."

It is fair to say, then, that social science is a macroscience that attempts to describe, measure, and predict attitudes and behaviors at the level of large groups or whole societies. The main purpose of social research is to categorize these attitudes, feelings, and behaviors to make inductive generalizations from a representative sample to a larger group, and the various social research methods and methodologies have been designed and developed largely with that purpose in mind.

When the research methods and methodologies of the social sciences were first introduced into the academic discipline of nursing in the 1960s and 1970s, it could be argued that they offered an appropriate paradigm for the profession. At that time, nursing care was usually organized and delivered in a task-centered way with a focus on finding the most efficient and effective means of providing routine and standardized care to large numbers of patients (Anderson, 1973). The Royal College of Nursing (1971) in the United Kingdom emphasized the nurse's role not in terms of a one-to-one relationship with patients but in reference to the nurse being a member of a group within society.

Research methods that provided statistical information about the general effectiveness of different approaches to various nursing tasks at the level of the group or society were therefore of great benefit in streamlining ward routines at a time when the completion of tasks often provided more satisfaction to nurses than patient-oriented goals (McLean, 1973).

It could be argued, however, that the academic discipline of nursing has failed to keep pace with subsequent changes to nursing practice. Since the introduction of the social science paradigm for the production and testing of nursing knowledge and theory, the focus of practice has shifted from the group to the individual. We can see this shift in the most recent definition of nursing from the RCN, which refers to caring for *"individuals* of all ages, families and communities, throughout the entire life span" and adds that

> the specific domain of nursing is people's *unique responses* to and experience of health, illness, frailty, disability and health related life events in whatever environment or circumstances they find themselves. (RCN, 2014, p. 3, emphasis added)

This represents a complete *volte-face* for the RCN from their earlier definition of nursing as a social activity and is echoed by the International Council of Nurses (ICN) in their statement that "nursing encompasses autonomous and collaborative care of *individuals* of all ages, families, groups and communities, sick or well and in all settings" (ICN, 2016, emphasis added).

It would seem, then, that academic nursing has not kept pace with the fundamental changes in the focus of practice. Although social research methods and methodologies might be appropriate for informing nursing policy and decisions at a macro level, they were never intended to tell us anything about what happens at the micro level of the unique therapeutic encounter between unique individuals in a unique setting at a unique moment in time. For this purpose, as we might expect, what is required is not a science of society informed by objective and generalizable research methodologies but *a science of the unique*, informed by methods and methodologies designed to provide individualized and contextualized knowledge that arises from and relates directly back to practice (Rolfe, 2006b; Rolfe 2015; Rolfe & Gardner, 2005).

NURSING AND EBP

Despite the argument for a more individualized approach, recent trends in nursing research appear to be moving in the very opposite direction. Nursing has for many years aspired to be recognized as a research-based profession, and as we have seen, this has generally been interpreted and understood in terms of the qualitative and quantitative methods and methodologies of the social science research paradigms. However, the past decade has increasingly witnessed a shift away from *research*-based practice toward EBP. On one level, this shift has been hardly noticeable, since many practitioners and some academics regard the two terms as more or less synonymous, often using the words *research* and *evidence* interchangeably. A closer examination of the tenets of EBP, however, reveals a clear bias toward evidence from experimental and quasi-experimental research studies and a subsequent shift from the social science research paradigms to the paradigms of medicine and agriculture.

Many advocates of EBP argue for a hierarchy in which the quality of the evidence is rated solely according to its method of production, and a number of hierarchies of evidence have been published over the past decade, all of which place evidence from randomized controlled trials (RCTs), and preferably evidence from systematic reviews of *several* RCTs, at the top (e.g., Evans, 2003; Thompson & Dowding, 2002).

The EBP movement clearly plays down the findings from nonexperimental social research, which is considered to be a lowly form of evidence and is only acceptable if it derives from more than one study by more than one research group. Although Polit and Beck (2014) suggest hopefully that "small studies designed to solve local problems will likely increase" (p. 4), such studies are unlikely to meet the strict criteria outlined previously. What is more likely, and is in fact already happening in the United Kingdom, is that research is becoming industrialized with large multidisciplinary teams conducting multimillion dollar production-line research projects with a division of labor in which each researcher has responsibility for only a small part of the research process and rarely gets an overview of the entire project. Nursing research is therefore becoming further removed from everyday practice and practitioners as small, individualized, and unfunded projects are being diminished in impact and importance.

However, the shift from research-based practice to EBP could be seen as far more dangerous and insidious than simply a scaling-up of research activity. I have already suggested that the social science research paradigms have located the focus of nursing research in the domain of knowledge and theory-testing rather than in practice, which in T. S. Eliot's phrase represents the loss of wisdom at the expense of knowledge. EBP, at least in its original and generally understood form, suggests a further shift in the focus of nursing research away from the traditional social science aim of *Verstehen* or understanding toward the scientific testing of nursing and medical interventions to produce "evidence" of their efficacy. The EBP movement has little regard for the building or testing of theory and is concerned primarily with effectiveness and efficiency; it is interested less in developing a coherent body of professional knowledge than in presenting an atheoretical patchwork of "experimentally tested" interventions. In T. S. Eliot's term, this represents the loss of knowledge in favor of information.

CHALLENGES TO THE HIERARCHY OF EVIDENCE

I suggested in the introduction to this chapter that the descent from wisdom to knowledge and to information entails a loss that cannot be retrieved. Wisdom can be reduced to knowledge but knowledge alone cannot be used to reconstitute that wisdom. Similarly, knowledge can be reduced to information, but information alone cannot be used to reconstruct knowledge. From this perspective, the data generated by RCTs might well offer practitioners reliable and valid information about the effectiveness of various nursing interventions, but it cannot provide them with the clinical wisdom necessary to make judicious decisions about the application of that information. Seen from this perspective, the findings from RCTs are of limited use to the practicing nurse; they provide the nurse with general population-level data that might or might not be taken into consideration as background information for clinical decisions, but they do not help in making the on-the-spot clinical judgments demanded of the wise practitioner.

Given that RCTs are located at the apex of most hierarchies of evidence, this is, perhaps, a surprising claim that requires further examination. The RCT, which is the foundation of EBP, is widely acknowledged as having its origins in agricultural research (Fisher, 1935), where it was developed as a means of comparing the effectiveness of pesticides or fertilizers on identical fields of crops. In its original format, then, the outcome measure of the RCT was overall crop yield, and the fate of individual plants was largely irrelevant. The RCT methodology was later applied to medicine, usually to test the efficacy and safety of newly developed drugs. Similarly, the outcome measure was usually taken to be overall clinical improvement or lessening of side effects in the experimental group when compared with a control group.

Clearly, the transition from agriculture to medicine entailed a number of modifications to the methodology. First, of course, medical researchers could not neglect the welfare of the individual; although it did not matter whether individual plants in the experimental group died, so long as there was an increase in overall yield, the same attitude could not be taken with human subjects in a drug trial. Second, refinements such as double blinds had to be introduced in recognition of some fundamental differences between plants and sentient humans. However, the methodology remained essentially the same: A treatment was considered to be more effective if the group of subjects to whom it was administered responded better than the group who received a placebo.

In cases where the treatment intervention is a drug or a medical procedure, the logic of the clinical trial is more or less sound: If a carefully selected and representative sample from a particular population responds to the intervention, then we can say with some statistical level of certainty that the entire population from which the sample was drawn will respond in a similar manner. What the trial does not enable us to do, however, is to make predictions about individual members of the population or about the effectiveness of the treatment in other contexts and settings. In the case of crop treatments or medical drugs, that hardly matters, since the assumption is that all members of the population will respond in much the same way regardless of the social, temporal, or physical context in which the treatment is administered (although, of course, the introduction of the double blind is a tacit acknowledgement of a social or psychological factor in physical responses to medicines). However, I have argued previously that clinical nursing practice is composed of a series of personal and unique interventions whose outcome will depend on a large number of social and contextual factors; indeed, that these social and contextual factors are sometimes of greater relevance to the outcome than the treatment itself. For the nurse, then, *information* about the average response to a nursing intervention by the population as a whole will not readily translate into *knowledge* about the idiosyncratic responses of individual patients or into clinical *wisdom* about whether to employ a particular intervention in a particular case with a particular patient in a particular setting at a particular time.

I am arguing that the hierarchy of evidence, with RCTs at its pinnacle and nonexperimental studies and experiential knowledge at the bottom, does not reflect the important and fundamental differences between the practice of medicine and the practice of nursing. A number of writers have responded to this discrepancy by proposing a new conceptualization of evidence-based *nursing* that takes into account the specific demands of the discipline. For example, Mulhall (1998) argued that "tiptoeing in the wake of the movement for evidence based medicine, we must ensure that evidence based nursing attends to what is important for nursing" (p. 4) and suggested that evidence from qualitative studies should be given equal status to evidence from RCTs. However, while a paradigm of evidence-based *nursing* might replace the RCT with qualitative methodologies at the apex of the hierarchy of evidence, such an approach nevertheless maintains and reinforces the separation between research and practice and between researchers and practitioners.

EBP AND TECHNICAL RATIONALITY

I wish to suggest, however, that the problem for nursing practice is deeper and more complex than simply a dispute over quantitative, qualitative, or (more recently) mixed-method approaches to the generation of research evidence. As I argued earlier, the issue is not so much a question of what kind of research evidence should form the basis of nursing practice but rather the very idea that nursing should be *based* on research evidence at all. Although this might appear to be a somewhat perverse claim, the question of what it means to base practice on research evidence is complex and pivotal to EBP but has been largely avoided by advocates of the EBP movement.

The original prospectus for EBP, as set out by the Evidence-Based Medicine Working Group (Guyatt et al., 1992), claimed that "evidence-based medicine de-emphasizes intuition [and] unsystematic clinical experience . . . and stresses the examination of evidence from clinical research" (p. 2420), specifically the RCT. Little was said about how the evidence was to be implemented, although Sackett, Rosenberg, Gray, Haynes, and Richardson (1996) later added that the practice of evidence-based medicine somehow entailed "integrating individual clinical expertise with the best available external clinical evidence from systematic research" (p. 71).

Precisely how individual clinical expertise and generalizable scientific research findings were to be integrated was never made clear, although Sackett et al. (1996) instructed that the clinical judgments of individual practitioners should always take precedence over research evidence. Presumably, these clinical judgments are based on the very same "unsystematic clinical experience" that the Evidence-Based Medicine Working Group claimed should be "de-emphasized," and it is difficult to conceptualize a model of EBP in which the evidence from "gold standard" research findings can, at any time, be overthrown by the unsystematic and unscientific judgments of the practitioner. Perhaps for these reasons, advocates of evidence-based approaches have tended to focus almost exclusively on the concept of *evidence* and have neglected to explore the equally important but vague and undertheorized notion of what it means to *base* practice on evidence.

When nurse academics first began to explore the possibilities for EBP in nursing, they imported the medical version more or less wholesale, retaining not only the importance of systematic research based on scientific rigor but also the emphasis on the concept of "evidence" and the relative neglect of the second word in the phrase *evidence-based practice*. So, for example, French (1998) defined EBP in nursing as "the process of systematic identification, rigorous evaluation and the subsequent dissemination and use of the findings of research to influence clinical practice" (p. 47).

While she identified "evidence" as the identification, evaluation, and dissemination of research findings, with the "gold standard" being the RCT, little consideration was given to how, in her words, evidence might *influence* clinical practice; that is, to what it means for practice to be *based* on evidence from research. Indeed, the translation of evidence into practice has usually been considered so straightforward as to barely merit a mention.

Although this might perhaps be the case in many medical settings, where EBP could mean simply the prescription of a drug or treatment regime that a clinical trial has shown to be effective, I have suggested that nursing practice is somewhat more complex and individualized. If evidence-based nursing is to have any authentic practical meaning, our definition of the concept of what might count as best evidence will be secondary to and dependent on what, if anything, it means for nursing practice to be *based* on evidence.

BEYOND TECHNICAL RATIONALITY

We can see that the word *based* acts here as a conjunctive, a word that serves to join the two separate and disparate activities of doing research and doing practice, thereby reinforcing the hierarchy advocated by technical rationality: Research and practice are linked in a causal relationship in which research activity determines evidence and evidence determines nursing practice. Rather than simply replace one research methodology with another at the top of a hierarchy of nursing evidence, I wish to advocate the radical approach of abandoning technical rationality altogether as the dominant paradigm for nursing practice. In other words, I want to propose an approach to doing nursing that is not *based* on evidence from externally conducted research but which integrates the collection and application of evidence into the practice of nursing itself.

If nursing practice is thought of as a series of unique encounters between individuals, then information about what tends to happen *in the average case* will be of limited use in making wise judgments about what to do *in any particular case*. Indeed, it could be argued that the only research findings that will be of any immediate practical use are those that arise from the specific case itself. This suggests that we should value and prioritize research evidence in nursing *not* according to whether it has been generated by the application of a rigorous, objective, controlled, decontextualized, and generalizable "scientific" methodology such as the RCT but by the extent to which it will be of benefit to the specific clinical situation in which the nurse currently finds herself. Generalized macro-level information might be of some limited use in discerning trends and possibilities, but the most important and valuable knowledge required by a nurse who needs to make a wise clinical decision *here and now with this unique individual patient* is the rich, contextualized knowledge that arises from the situation itself during the course of the clinical encounter.

It follows that the person best placed to conduct research into specific clinical nurse–patient encounters is the nurse (or, in certain cases, the patient). The most important and useful research methodologies for a science of the unique are therefore those that incorporate practitioner research in which nurses conduct on-the-spot inquiry into their own practice. Furthermore, the findings from practitioner research do not have to be written up and published before they can be applied to practice but have the potential immediately to influence the clinical encounter from which they originated. A science of the unique is therefore an immediate and fully *reflexive* one that unites research and practice (and also researcher and practitioner) in the integrated act of *praxis* and results in wise action based on an intimate, rich, and contextual experiential knowledge of unique individual cases.

The rejection of technical rationality in favor of praxis does not merely *call into question* the relationship between the researcher and the practitioner; rather, it completely dissolves the distinction between them. Praxis is a form of on-the-spot experimentation that attempts to integrate research, theorizing, and practice into a single activity to be carried out by a practitioner–researcher in the clinical area. As such, it stands outside the mainstream of both the social science and the medical paradigms and draws on the traditions and epistemologies of more established practice disciplines such as education, psychotherapy, and political science. We can hear echoes in praxis of Karl Marx's dictum that "the philosophers have only interpreted the world, in various ways; the point is to change it" (Marx, 1845/1970, p. 123) and of Kurt Lewin's admonition that "research that produces nothing but books will not suffice" (Lewin, 1948, p. 203). The epistemology underpinning praxis is perhaps most succinctly summed up by Peter Reason under the rubric of "co-operative inquiry," which

> seeks knowledge in action for action. Co-operative researchers may write books and articles, but often the knowledge that is really important for them is the practical knowledge of new skills and abilities. . . . And thus in co-operative inquiry,

education and social action may become fully integrated with the research process. (Reason, 1988, p. 13)

As Reason points out, the *process* involved in doing this type of research might include education and social action as well as data collection and therefore takes on a significance and importance far beyond what would be expected in traditional technical rational methodologies. In addition, the *outcome* is far wider in scope than mere books and articles, which, as Lewin tells us, simply will not do. The aims of praxis are *practical knowledge* and *practical change* for both the nurse *and* the patient.

This is not intended to be a methods chapter, and, in any case, praxis is not defined by the data collection methods it employs, which can be many and varied (including quantitative methods) and which are chosen pragmatically to suit the task in hand. There are, however, a number of methodological approaches that are particularly suited to the aims of praxis, and these include participative and emancipatory action research, reflexive ethnography, single-case experiments, cooperative inquiry, and some approaches to reflective and reflexive practice. These methodologies share a number of features that make them particularly useful for nurses who wish to explore and improve their practice.

TOWARD SOME METHODOLOGICAL PRINCIPLES OF PRAXIS

1. Praxis, as we have seen, is a science of the unique and takes as its starting point the observation by the poet W. H. Auden (1967/1990) that "as persons, we are incomparable, unclassifiable, uncountable, irreplaceable" (p. 6). Thus, *praxis is a science of individual persons rather than a science of people as a collective whole.* I have argued previously that while many of the qualitative social science methodologies purport to study individuals, most are concerned ultimately with generalizing or categorizing the findings to a wider population (statistical generalization) or to a general theory (analytic generalization). The methodologies employed in praxis are concerned primarily with unique individual cases, and no attempt is made to move from the specific to the general. We can see this approach, for example, in single-case experiments, which use mostly quantitative data collection methods to explore the effects of particular treatment or caring interventions on specific individual patients. Through careful pre- and posttesting, nurses are able to measure and modify the effects of their own interventions over time and thus to tailor individual care to meet the needs of their unique and individual patients. The purpose of single-case experiments

is to learn about the unique needs and responses of individuals, and no attempt is made to generalize or transfer the findings between patients.

2. *Praxis places the practitioner–researcher at the heart of the research process.* Whereas many social and medical research methodologies could be described as practitioner based, insofar as they include practitioners in the research process, perhaps collecting data or administering treatment interventions, praxis methodologies all involve the practitioner–researcher in the critical analysis of some aspect of the nurse's own practice. Praxis methodologies are therefore not merely practitioner *based* but might be better described as practitioner *centered*. The most fundamental and straightforward practitioner-centered research methodology is what Schön (1983) described as reflection-on-action, which entails a systematic and critical approach to thinking and writing about and learning from our own practice and, most importantly, applying what has been learned back into practice at the earliest opportunity.

3. We can see, then, that *praxis entails not only reflectivity but also reflexivity,* the application of research findings back into the practice setting from which they were gathered by the practitioner–researcher who gathered them. Reflexivity can be seen most clearly and overtly in Schön's (1983) other strategy for reflection, which he called reflection-*in*-action or on-the-spot experimenting. Reflection-in-action, in its most advanced form, involves a cyclical process of assessing the current situation, formulating a hypothesis, testing it through practical interventions, and reevaluating the situation in the light of the intervention (Schön, 1983). This experimental cycle is conducted in the midst of practice by the practitioner–researcher as part of everyday *modus operandi*; it is, at the same time, a way of doing research and a way of doing nursing. As a cyclical process, reflection-in-action is both continuous (one cycle leads inexorably to the next) and continual (unlike most research methodologies, it has no termination point, for example, when the funding runs out). Reflection-in-action might therefore be regarded as the most fundamental and widely used methodology of praxis.

4. *The experimental approach described previously is common to all of the methodologies employed in praxis.* For example, action research, as originally defined by Lewin (1948), "proceeds in a series of steps each of which is composed of a circle of planning, action, and fact-finding about the result of the action" (p. 206). In all cases, practitioner–researchers experiment with their practice by conducting a series of *systematic* and *controlled* treatment or caring interventions, which are then modified or revised according to what Lewin referred to as "fact-finding about the result of the action."

5. While all practitioner-centered research is systematic and controlled, practitioner–researchers would generally reject the criterion of rigor that is much favored by social researchers. We have already seen that, in most social research

methodologies, validity and reliability are guaranteed by rigorous adherence to method; in other words, the findings are to be trusted if and only if the prescribed method can be shown to have been followed rigorously and unswervingly. Practitioner research, however, is concerned less with valid and reliable findings than with positive action, and positive action depends on the reflexivity of the practitioner–researcher in responding to feedback as it arises. Whereas rigor implies rigidity and rule-following, *practitioner–researchers will value flexibility and rule bending (and, at times, rule breaking)*. See, for example, Rolfe (2006a) for an account of research validity based on Lyotard's idea of rule-free judgments.

6.   Finally, and perhaps most controversially, *practitioner–researchers reject the objective stance of the disinterested researcher.* They neither step back so as not to influence the "objects" of their research nor "bracket" their own preconceptions and leave them at the door. For example, cooperative inquirers actively engage with their "subjects" as partners in the research process and are thus fully immersed in the practice being studied. Stenhouse (1981) described the stance of the practitioner–researcher as "interested," not only in the sense of taking an interest in the issues and practices being researched but also in the sense of having a vested interest in the outcome of the research. Gadamer (1976) referred to this stance more straightforwardly as "prejudice" and regarded it not only as unavoidable but also as advantageous to the researcher. As Stenhouse argued, the first and foremost reason for conducting research into our own practice is to make things better, and we therefore have to exercise our professional judgment as to what constitutes improvement. For the practitioner–researcher, there is no objective, value-neutral viewpoint "out there" from which to conduct research. Like it or not, the nurse is fully immersed in the research-practice experience.

CONCLUSIONS

A number of writers have commented over the years on the existence of the so-called "theory–practice gap" in nursing. The blame for this gap between what theorists and researchers state *should* happen in practice and what *actually* happens is usually laid firmly at the feet of practitioners for not reading, understanding, and implementing the latest research findings. In this chapter, I have turned the tables by suggesting that the problem lies less with practice than with research, that the dominant nursing research methods and methodologies have not kept pace with changes in nursing practice, and that, subsequently, neither the methodologies themselves nor the findings derived from those methodologies are fit for the purpose of informing practicing nurses in the 21st century. I have further suggested that what is required is not simply a reconsideration and revision of the so-called "hierarchy of evidence" but rather a radical review of the technical rational relationship between research and practice.

The traditional technical rational paradigm of EBP regards research and clinical nursing as two separate and distinct activities, while generally failing to explicate in any detail just what links them, that is, what it might mean in practical terms for a nurse to *base* practice on the findings of large-scale statistical research. Rather than merely *basing* practice on research evidence, I have proposed a new epistemology of praxis that fully *integrates* the activities of research gathering and nursing practice into a single, seamless activity undertaken by a single person, in which research and practice are constantly informing and responding to one another.

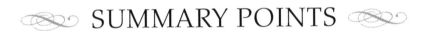

SUMMARY POINTS

1. Nursing requires an approach to knowledge and knowledge development substantially and distinctly different from that used in medical and social sciences.

2. The tenets of EBP are more congruent with the hierarchy of knowledge promoted by its originating sciences, medicine, and agriculture, rather than with nursing's individualized approach to the unique and complex needs of patients.

3. A *science of the unique person* is proposed, which promotes praxis over technical rationality and can seamlessly combine practice and research to produce knowledge and wisdom for nursing practice.

4. A *science of the unique* involves an immediate and fully *reflexive* approach that unites research and practice (and also the researcher and the practitioner) in the integrated act of *praxis* and results in wise action based on an intimate, rich, and contextual experiential knowledge of unique individual cases.

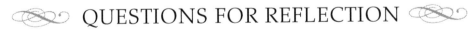 QUESTIONS FOR REFLECTION

1. Think about your own understanding of the term *evidence-based nursing.* What do you consider to be the most useful and valuable sources of evidence for your own practice? What is it about these sources of evidence that makes them more useful to you?

2. Think of a recent case where you applied evidence in making a clinical, managerial, or other person-centered decision. Reflect on what was going

through your mind as you weighed up the various pieces of evidence that contributed to your decision.

3. Think about some of the implications for practice and research of adopting a research paradigm based on a science of individual persons rather than collectively on people. How would the practices of nursing and research differ from the current paradigm? In particular, what would be the implications for patients of this new way of working?

❧ REFERENCES ❧

Anderson, E. R. (1973). *The role of the nurse.* London, England: Royal College of Nursing.

Auden, W. H. (1990). A short defense of poetry. In M. van Manen (Ed.), *Researching lived experience* (p. 6). New York, NY: SUNY. (Original work published 1967)

Eliot, T. S. (1940). The rock. In T. S. Eliot (Ed.), *Collected poems* (pp. 107–127). London, England: Faber and Faber. (Original work published 1934)

Evans, D. (2003) Hierarchy of evidence: A framework for ranking evidence evaluating healthcare interventions. *Journal of Clinical Nursing, 12,* 77–84.

Fisher, R. A. (1935). *The design of experiments.* Edinburgh, United Kingdom: Oliver and Boyd.

French, B. (1998). Developing the skills required for evidence-based practice. *Nurse Education Today, 18,* 46–51.

Gadamer, H. G. (1976). *Philosophical hermeneutics.* Berkeley: University of California Press.

Giddens, A., & Sutton, P. W. (2013). *Sociology* (7th ed.). Cambridge, United Kingdom: Polity Press.

Greenwood, E. (1966). Attributes of a profession. In H. M. Vollmer & D. L. Mills (Eds.), *Professionalization* (pp. 10–19). Englewood Cliffs, NJ: Prentice-Hall.

Guyatt, G., Cairns, J., Churchill, D., Cook, D., Haynes, B., Hirsh, J., . . . Tugwell, P. (1992). Evidence-based medicine: A new approach to teaching the practice of medicine. *Journal of the American Medical Association, 268,* 2420–2425.

Hammersley, M., & Atkinson, P. (2007). *Ethnography: Principles in practice* (3rd ed.). London, England: Routledge.

International Council of Nurses. (2016). Definition of nursing. Retrieved from http://www.icn.ch/about-icn/icn-definition-of-nursing

Kalisch, P. A., & Kalisch, B. J. (2004). *The advance of American nursing: A history* (4th ed.). Philadelphia, PA: J. B. Lippincott.

Lewin, K. (1948). Action research and minority problems. In G. W. Lewin (Ed.), *Resolving social conflicts: Selected papers on group dynamics* (pp. 201–216). New York, NY: Harper & Row.

Marx, K. (1970). Theses on Feuerbach. In K. Marx, F. Engels (Eds.), & C. J. Arthur (Trans.), *The German ideology* (pp. 121–123). London, England: Lawrence & Wishart. (Original work published 1845)

McLean, J. P. (1973). Nursing care study: Bilateral nephrectomy. *Nursing Mirror, 136*(10), 31–34.

Mulhall, A. (1998). Nursing, research and the evidence. *Evidence-Based Nursing, 1*(1), 4–6.

Nightingale, F. (1860). *Notes on nursing: What it is, and what it is not.* New York, NY: D. Appleton.

Polit, D. E., & Beck, C. T. (2004). *Nursing research: Principles and methods* (7th ed.). Philadelphia, PA: Lippincott Williams & Wilkins.

Polit, D. E., & Beck, C. T. (2006). *Essentials of nursing research: Methods, appraisal, and utilization* (6th ed.). Philadelphia, PA: Lippincott Williams & Wilkins.

Polit, D. E., & Beck, C. T. (2014). *Essentials of nursing research: Appraising evidence for nursing practice* (8th ed.). Philadelphia, PA: Lippincott Williams & Wilkins.

Polit, D. E., & Beck, C. T. (2017). *Nursing research: Generating and assessing evidence for nursing practice* (10th ed.). Philadelphia, PA: Lippincott Williams & Wilkins.

Priyjmachuk, S. (1996). A nursing perspective on the interrelationships between theory, research and practice. *Journal of Advanced Nursing, 23,* 679–684.

Reason, P. (1988). *Human inquiry in action.* London, England: Sage.

Rolfe, G. (2006a). Judgments without rules: Towards a postmodern ironist concept of research validity. *Nursing Inquiry, 13,* 7–15.

Rolfe, G. (2006b). Nursing praxis and the science of the unique. *Nursing Science Quarterly, 19*(1), 39–43.

Rolfe, G. (2015). Foundations for a human science of nursing: Gadamer, Laing, and the hermeneutics of caring. *Nursing Philosophy, 16*(3), 141–152.

Rolfe, G., & Gardner, L. (2005). Towards a nursing science of the unique: Evidence, reflexivity and the study of persons. *Journal of Research in Nursing, 10,* 297–310.

Royal College of Nursing. (1971). *Evidence to the Committee on Nursing.* London, England: Author.

Sackett, D. L., Rosenberg, W. M. C., Gray, J. A. M., Haynes, R. B., & Richardson, W. S. (1996). Evidence based medicine: What it is and what it isn't. *British Journal of Medicine, 312,* 71–72.

Schön, D. (1983). *The reflective practitioner.* London, England: Temple Smith.

Stenhouse, L. (1978). Case study and case records: Towards a contemporary history of education. *British Educational Research Journal, 4*(2), 21–39.

Stenhouse, L. (1981). What counts as research? *British Journal of Educational Studies, 29*(2), 103–114.

Thompson, C., & Dowding, D. (2002). *Clinical decision making and judgement in nursing.* Edinburgh, Scotland: Churchill Livingstone.

5

Interlude I: *The Mandala and Discovering Nursing Worldviews*

Nelma B. Crawford Shearer

Doctorally prepared nurses in practice play a significant role in advancing the production of nursing knowledge. They have not only clinical expertise, but also a repertoire of patient-practice experiences that serve as a source in developing knowledge, particularly nursing theory. Although clinical practice "is the field for knowledge development" (Arslanian-Engoren, Hicks, Whall, & Algase, 2005, p. 317), coursework helps students clarify philosophical perspectives about nursing that are useful in developing one's skills in knowledge production. "Practice is not a 'stand alone' phenomenon" but is an outcome of philosophical beliefs and values (Whall, 2005, p. 1). What is often neglected in theory development to guide interventions is the conceptual work to clarify the nurse's philosophical views and beliefs and concepts of interest that feed the synergy for knowledge between practice and theoretical thinking.

Given the fact that our philosophical views pervade our practice and research, whether we are fully aware of it or not, it is advantageous to take a few moments to consider just what are our philosophical views about relevant concepts like health, human beings, environment, and nursing. This can be done by exploring nursing worldviews. Clarifying one's own worldview is one of the first steps in developing as a scholar and contributor to nursing knowledge. Philosophical views are a pathway to inform ethical practice and to stimulate conceptual ideas. In this *interlude*, I present a strategy to help students learn about and articulate philosophical views underlying nursing activities in practice, education, and research.

Nurses engage in what I call *theorizing on their feet* when they integrate theoretical thinking with their practice experiences. This happens more than we may realize. However, historically and still now, theory and practice are regarded as two separate processes. The literature is replete with examples of this, and it is reflected in students' emails, such as, "I'm spending more time on this class than any other class. Theory is important to nursing, but I think that I need to spend more time on health assessment and pathophysiology." Nevertheless, I am pleased that students challenge the importance of philosophy and theory in nursing. So to meet this challenge, I developed a teaching strategy to take my students on a journey designed to engage them in theoretical thinking, specifically to clarify their philosophical perspectives about nursing as they look through and perhaps even refocus their practice lens.

LET THE JOURNEY BEGIN

As with all journeys, learning to "theorize on your feet" begins with foundational steps. One way to begin is with a theory class assignment to help students describe and ponder the role of nursing science (Barrett, 2002) or debate the purpose of nursing theory in practice (Cody, 2003). These kinds of readings introduce elements that comprise nursing's structure of knowledge including worldviews, the nursing metaparadigm, and theories. The readings are also useful in exploring the relationships among abstract terms like *science, practice, research,* and *theory.* But perhaps the most important assignment, once students have knowledge of what some of the experts say about nursing science and theory, is for students to consider their *own* expertise and to reflect on the ideas they cherish in nursing.

Using ideas from the readings and reflections on practice, I invite students to discuss a few deceptively simple questions drawn from the readings and posted on our online discussion board: "What is the focus of our discipline?" "When you walk into your patient's room, what do you first observe and assess?" "Why?" With a little coaching, students notice that their responses to the first question may reflect our nursing metaparadigm concepts: health, person, environment, nursing practice. Or students may discover other key concepts not yet considered as part of the nursing metaparadigm. Responses to the second question often address technology and the machines hooked up to the patient. During the online discussion, one doctoral student began to question her perception of the patient for whom she most recently provided care. "As I look back on the past few weeks," she reflected,

> I am trying to remember if I viewed my patient and/or their family as a whole, instead of their parts. I think it's easy to get caught up in taking care of a patient from a physiological perspective and not remembering the person has thoughts, feelings, and is part of a family.

These discussions of the readings, informed by students' practice experiences, serve as a catalyst to spark creativity in thinking theoretically as well as philosophically; that is, to think about their interest area for inquiry and then to delve deeper into the *why* behind their interests or what worldviews influence their thinking.

WORLDVIEWS IN NURSING

A worldview or paradigm reflects the discipline as a whole and the subject matter addressed by the discipline. A worldview seeks to answer two types of philosophical issues: views of reality (ontology) and views of knowledge (epistemology; Arslanian-Engoren et al., 2005; Polifroni, 2015).

Several philosophical perspectives have been offered by nursing scholars. Newman, Sime, and Corcoran-Perry (1991) offer three perspectives on nursing theory and the development of practice knowledge: the particulate-deterministic, the interactive-integrative, and the unitary-transformative. From an analysis of these and other worldviews, Fawcett (1993, 2005) arrived at her synthesis of the worldviews into three parts: reaction, reciprocal-interaction, and simultaneous action.

A nurse practicing from the *particulate-deterministic* or *reaction* perspective regards phenomena as reducible, and with fully definable properties that are orderly and predictably connected to one another. Change is viewed as something that can be controlled. Human beings are viewed as a composite of parts, as biopsychosocial-spiritual beings. The metaphor for human beings is the "machine" (Reed, 1995).

The *interactive-integrative* or *reciprocal-interaction* perspective presents phenomena as having multiple interrelated parts and change as a function of multiple factors and probabilistic relationships (Fawcett, 1993, 2005; Newman et al., 1991). Human beings are viewed as holistic, with parts understood within the context of the whole. Human beings are active, acting upon a passive environment. The biological organism is the metaphor for human beings (Reed, 1995).

From the *unitary-transformative* or *simultaneous-action* perspective, the nurse views phenomena as unitary, self-organizing, identified by pattern, and in process with the environment (Fawcett, 1993, 2005; Newman et al., 1991). Change in human beings and their environment is ongoing and unpredictable. The historical event (with the person as embedded in ongoing change and a historical context) is the metaphor for human beings (Reed, 1995).

PHILOSOPHICAL VIEW

Perhaps because of their perceived lack of familiarity with the theory dimension of their science, doctoral nursing students are eager to find ways to bring conceptual ideas, including their own philosophic views, to the forefront of their practice. They know that theory is a source of knowledge for improving patient care while optimizing patient health. However, theory and theorizing may provide little meaning until theory is personalized. It was time to refocus my lens! I endeavored to expand my more traditional approach of teaching nursing theory, through reading and discussion activities, to an approach that highlighted and captured students' creative processes. So I designed a learning experience involving drawing a mandala to help students begin to personalize the theory process, beginning with their own broad philosophical ideas. This mandala drawing activity helps students elucidate new meanings and organize their ideas as they grapple with nursing theory and knowledge production, particularly as related to their practice experiences.

ROLE OF THE MANDALA IN CLARIFYING YOUR WORLDVIEW

The word *mandala* comes from the classical Indian language of Sanskrit and means "circle" (The Mandala Project, n.d.). The circular shape signifies wholeness and can be viewed as an organizing framework with a unifying center. Mandalas contain symbols and patterns regarding all aspects of life and nature, such as in Earth and the sun, a flower, or a snowflake. The mandala is also used to depict a circle of life, including a community of friends and family. The mandala pattern is visible in certain cultures and religious traditions, as well as in architecture. For example, American Indians have used a circular shape to create the medicine wheel, whereas religious groups create circles or labyrinths for meditation and architects design structures built around a center.

Because a mandala contains symbols and patterns that are personally meaningful to nurses, creating a mandala may increase awareness of and thinking about values and beliefs—that is, philosophical views—that influence practice and research. A self-exploration as framed within a mandala provides insight into the nursing perspectives that are translated into daily nursing practice.

SELF-EXPLORATION

To initiate self-exploration, put this book down for a moment and reflect on your practice experiences and readings on theory and research literature. Think of strategies you might use to relax and open up to new ideas. For example, enjoy a walk, sit outside and relish the cool breeze of the early morning or late afternoon, take a swim, find a quiet place inside or outside under a tree, or listen to some music. Next, view the world as a mandala: a circle with a unifying center. Incorporate visual cues from nature with your nursing practice experiences and begin to create a mandala of nursing's metaparadigm: person, environment, health, and nurse.

Questions to guide this reflection are as follows: "What is the focal point of my mental picture?" "Is it the patient, nurse, health, environment, or something else?"

From there, draw the picture that is in your mind on a piece of paper or go to your computer and recreate your mental picture. If you are having trouble creating your picture, let the idea of a mandala or circle assist you in turning your visualization into a picture. Look at your drawing and think about your practice; what is the organizing framework and unifying center? Is person, nurse, health, or environment at the center of your practice? Step back and reflect on your drawing as you have produced a creative vision of your everyday practice. "How do you define or characterize these broad concepts?" Now think about your worldview or your philosophical perspective of nursing. "Do you view people as machines, as biological organisms, or from a developmental, historical perspective?" Think about your practice experiences: "What is the unifying center of your practice experiences?"

Description of Mandala (Figure 5.1)

Person (composed of roots and plant): I represented the *person* with a plant. It is divided in two specific ways, particularly in its interaction with the environment (the plant portion) and the nursing (the root portion). Together they make up one full person (dandelion) and neither can exist without the other. I chose a dandelion because they are highly resilient, show distinct stages, and are common throughout the world. The plant is large to acknowledge the plant itself and its physical entity but also skewed to one side to equally incorporate the environmental, health, and nursing aspects of the individual, acknowledging that those factors highly influence the plant's overall health.

Environment (composed of wind and sun): The environment composes the *external forces* that both benefit and harm the life cycle. Both the wind and the sun represent necessary factors to allow growth and energy (sun providing energy) and progression (wind blowing seeds) in life.

Health (composed of seed and garden): This aspect of the metaparadigm incorporates the plant's *life progression and purpose for existence.* This includes the interpretations of the physical, cultural, and spiritual aspects of life. The progression of the plant (seed) signifies the plant's autonomy because only a healthy plant that exists harmoniously with the other three major categories will propagate and flourish amid a community (garden). This category further includes the person's views on normal health progression and life after death.

Nursing (composed of watering and gardening): This portion of the represented metaparadigm related the external aspects of natural watering and gardening and the spiritual/God influence on our lives. It is an action performed by any *intentional* external autonomous presence in order to benefit the health of the person. In this category, both the human and spiritual forces necessary and benefiting survival exist. Nursing involves caring, skill, and particular knowledge in taking care of the plant and its needs.

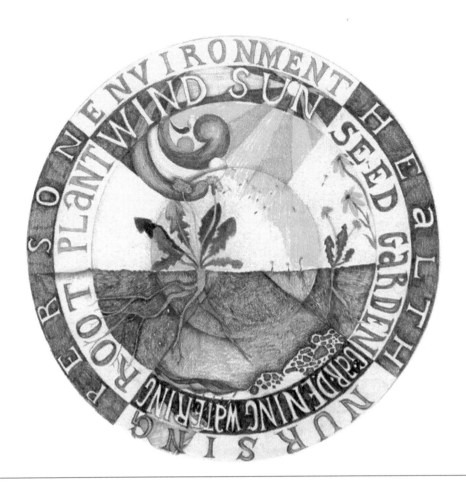

FIGURE 5.1 Mandala by Timothy Kruth.
Reprinted with permission by Timothy Kruth.

Description of Mandala (Figure 5.2)

Person-singular soul in universe, living spirit researching for soul enrichment through experience in life, conception, seed, egg, growth, and death complete the life circle of continuing human evolvement. Health obtained from harmony in living on the Earth and dreaming of the universe, progression obtained with well-being in existence. Seek pathway for continued well-being in existence. Environment-sun is source of energy for creation of life, Earth is provider of life energy with collaboration of sun's energy and Earth is mother for shelter and sustenance, the capsule of life suspended in the universe of unknowns. Nursing facilitates pathway creation for harmony in health and environment for person, to achieve balance in earthly existence, support dream of universe, and place in existence by promotion of love through caring.

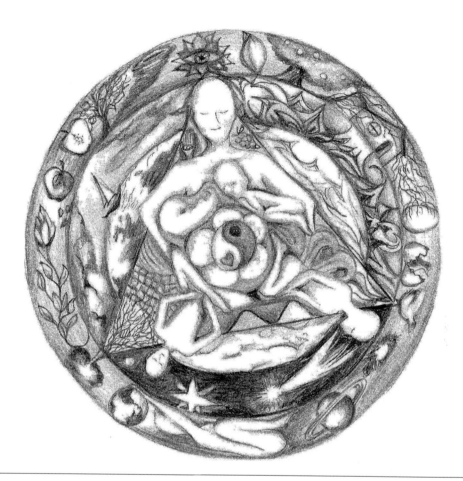

FIGURE 5.2 Mandala by Lisa Green.
Reprinted with permission by Lisa Green.

ARTICULATING A WORLDVIEW AS A LINK TO PRACTICE

Based on your worldview, the center of the drawing may consist of anything from stick figures to an elaborate drawing with the focal point of a patient, nurse, environment, or health. Regardless of the focal point, think about the center of your drawing and why you chose this as your focal point in relationship to worldviews in nursing.

Next, consider which nursing worldview your mandala most portrays. Do you perceive the patient and practice from the *particulate-deterministic* or *reaction* perspective worldview in which human beings are viewed as machines and health is viewed as a consequence of a single event? That is, do you emphasize a cause–effect relationship in which the patient returns to a state of equilibrium, with balance as the health goal? If this worldview is congruent with your perspective, you may view your role as developing a care plan for the patient who focuses on reducing personal risk for disease and death.

If your worldview is more in line with the *interactive-integrative* or *reciprocal-interaction* perspective, you perceive a human being as a living biological open system. Health and illness occur simultaneously within the human–environment relationship. In your practice, you center your attention on optimizing the patient's health while focusing on the patient rather than his or her environment.

The *unitary-transformative* or *simultaneous-action* worldview proposes that there are many ways of viewing and explaining health and the patient. If this worldview appears to be congruent with your perspective as reflected in your mandala, you may believe that health and illness occur simultaneously within the human–environment process and are not viewed as separate events. Changes in health occur through an interactive relationship with the environment, and are ongoing and irreversible, innovative, and developmental. You perceive the patient as interacting with the environment and recognize health as embedded in a context that changes from moment to moment. When practicing from this worldview, you focus on the patient as well as the patient's family and environment to optimize his or her well-being.

LET THE JOURNEY CONTINUE

Whether you realize it or not, you have begun the process of philosophical inquiry by clarifying some of your own beliefs and definitions about concepts basic to nursing. This in turn provides a personal foundation for making some of the choices you will face as a practitioner and knowledge-builder of nursing. Now, revisit philosophical inquiry questions intended to inspire your scientific inquiry in practice and research by asking yourself: "What is nursing?" "What are the elements of a human being that nursing should attend to?" "How do I define health, and is it ethical to apply my definition to patients?" These questions may never go away, and you may revisit them again and again as you pursue a scholarly career in nursing.

Regardless of where the process begins, self-exploration and articulating a worldview through a mandala is intended to enhance understanding of your own philosophy about human beings, health, nursing, and the environment—nursing's metaparadigm. In addition, your descriptions of the metaparadigm concepts provide a framework for recognizing your worldview of nursing and either refocusing or confirming your practice lens. Let the journey that began with self-exploration and culminated in the recognition of your worldview continue as you develop into a scholar and contributor to nursing knowledge.

SUMMARY POINTS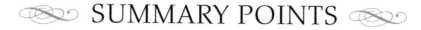

1. Nurses engage in *theorizing on their feet* when they integrate theoretical thinking with their practice experiences.

2. Philosophical inquiry begins by clarifying personal beliefs and definitions of nursing's metaparadigm.

3. Descriptions of human beings, health, nursing, and environment provide a framework for recognizing your worldview of nursing.

4. The process of drawing a mandala is a creative way to begin clarifying personal beliefs and definitions about concepts basic to nursing.

QUESTIONS FOR REFLECTION

1. Based on your drawing, what worldview or philosophical views seem congruent with your practice?

2. How has this chapter helped you refocus your practice lens?

3. Which of the mandalas presented here do you prefer and why, in terms of the philosophic views it conveys to you?

4. What role could recognizing your worldview play in your development as a scholar and contributor to nursing knowledge?

REFERENCES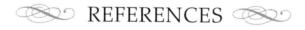

Arslanian-Engoren, C., Hicks, F. D., Whall, A. L., & Algase, D. L. (2005). An ontological view of advanced practice nursing. *Research and Theory for Nursing Practice, 19,* 315–322.

Barrett, E. A. M. (2002). What is nursing science? *Nursing Science Quarterly, 15*(1), 51–60.

Cody, W. K. (2003). Nursing theory as a guide to practice. *Nursing Science Quarterly, 16,* 225–231.

Fawcett, J. (1993). For a plethora of paradigms to parsimony in worldviews. *Nursing Science Quarterly, 6*(3), 56–59.

Fawcett, J. (2005). *Contemporary nursing knowledge: Analysis and evaluation of nursing models and theories* (2nd ed.). Philadelphia, PA: F. A. Davis.

The Mandala Project. (n.d.). What is a mandala? Retrieved from http://www.mandala project.org/what/index.html

Newman, M. A., Sime, A. M., & Corcoran-Perry, S. A. (1991). The focus of the discipline of nursing. *Advances in Nursing Science, 14*(1), 1–6.

Polifroni, E. C. (2015). Philosophy of science: An introduction. In J. B. Butts & K. L. Rich (Eds.), *Philosophies and theories for advanced nursing practice* (pp. 3–18). Burlington, MA: Jones & Bartlett.

Reed, P. G. (1995). A treatise on nursing knowledge development for the 21st century: Beyond postmodernism. *Advances in Nursing Science, 17*(3), 70–84.

Whall, A. L. (2005). "Lest we forget": An issue concerning the doctorate of nursing practice (DNP). *Nursing Outlook, 53*(1), 1.

The DNP Project: Translating Research Into Knowledge for Practice

Jennifer Ruel, Donna Behler McArthur, and Pamela G. Reed

The doctorate of nursing practice (DNP) degree, as the highest level of formal education for advanced nursing practice, presents a distinct opportunity to advance nursing knowledge. The evolution of the DNP degree has occurred within the context of burgeoning knowledge, changes in health care delivery, escalating demands of chronic illness care, diverse patient populations, and globalization. With DNP academic programs spanning every state in the nation, the potential impact of advanced practice doctorally prepared graduates on knowledge generation and health care outcomes is exponential. DNP-prepared nurses will have opportunities to transcend current barriers and affirmatively impact health care while bridging research and practice. A fundamental learning experience to equip nurses for these opportunities is the DNP project. The DNP project demonstrates synthesis of coursework, methods of inquiry, and practice in attaining *The Essentials of Doctoral Education for Advanced Practice Nursing* (American Association of College of Nursing [AACN], 2006). This chapter presents ideas to guide use of the DNP project as well as to sharpen thinking behind this innovative form of scholarly inquiry.

RESPONDING TO THE NEED FOR PRACTICE KNOWLEDGE

A hallmark of the practice doctorate is a program of study that develops clinical scholarship and practice expertise within the specialty as well as core knowledge regarding quality improvement (QI) initiatives (McArthur, 2017). Development of practice expertise begins as the DNP student acquires current clinical competencies and preparation for the ever-changing health care system. In addition, the DNP project provides students with opportunities to develop clinical scholarship by applying the tools and knowledge acquired through their education for knowledge innovation needed in 21st century health care.

The DNP project presents challenges as well as opportunities for educators and students. For example, depending on the student's point of entry into the academic program (BSN to DNP or MSN to DNP), his or her clinical experience and expertise may influence what resources he or she has for generating research questions and for collaborating with practice partners, agencies, and organizations. Also, research results indicate that the design, development, and implementation of the DNP project may vary across educational settings and require continued refinement (Auerbach et al., 2014; Dols, Hernández, & Miles, 2017). Nevertheless, the DNP project is a scholarly process that provides students the opportunity to engage in practice-relevant research.

Within the past decade there has been a paradigm shift in doctoral education in nursing (M. A. Brown & Crabtree, 2013). A major goal of the practice doctorate is to reduce the time lag between the discovery of knowledge and its implementation in practice to enhance health care providers' local practice knowledge. In keeping with this goal, the results from DNP projects and DNP graduates' research typically are not universally generalizable in the positivist sense of science; practitioners generate new knowledge transferable to practice. This is so in part because of the research design, attention to stakeholders, and accounting for contextual factors as well as existing evidence. Knowledge developed by the DNP-prepared nurse contributes to improved outcomes by the transferability of findings generated through practice-relevant research. Indeed, research conducted by PhD students often is not generalizable. Rather than draw distinctions between PhD and DNP doctoral research projects that may diminish the significance of one over the other, both must be regarded as building capacity for nursing knowledge.

In 2006, AACN described the DNP project as a specific project that demonstrates synthesis of the student's work and lays the foundation for future scholarship. In August 2015, the AACN DNP Task Force made new recommendations regarding the DNP project (AACN, 2015). Recommendations include a focus on a change that impacts health care outcomes through direct or indirect care; a systems or population/aggregate approach; demonstration of implementation; a plan for sustainability; an evaluation of process or outcomes; and a foundation for future practice scholarship.

KNOWLEDGE TRANSLATION AND THE DNP

Helping students discern both the distinction and synergy between evidence-based practice and the translation of research findings and best evidence into practice is an important component of educating students into the scholarship of their DNP role. Evidence-based practice requires, in the first place, research findings to generate evidence that informs practice. The subsequent translation of these research findings into sustainable improvements in clinical practice and patient outcomes is directly related to improved quality of health care (Agency for Healthcare Research & Quality, 2001).

Clearly there is a global health care system challenge—improving quality of care and outcomes, while decreasing adverse effects. Translating research into knowledge for practice addresses these challenges through approaches to inquiry, such as those modeled in the DNP project, that more actively link research and practice. Research evidence alone is insufficient for effective nursing practice. *Knowledge translation* addresses these challenges because it engages, in an iterative way, many resources including patient and family knowledge and values, other stakeholders, contextual factors, and nurses' expertise and patterns of knowing in translating research knowledge for practice (see Table 6.1).

Evidence-based practice integrates knowledge from Carper's (1978) four domains: empirics, aesthetics, personal knowledge, and ethics. The DNP student and graduate integrates the scientific knowledge of human behavior in health and illness, the aesthetic perception of significant human experiences, a personal understanding of the unique individuality of the self, and the capacity to make choices within concrete situations involving particular moral judgments. All domains inform the DNP project and are included in the knowledge translation process for evidence-based practice.

The knowledge translation process associated with the DNP project is but one of various approaches to reducing the time lag between knowledge discovery and implementation. For example, there are programs of research based on theories and methods (e.g., Kitson, Harvey, & McCormack [1998], Kitson & Harvey [2016], and Rycroft-Malone et al. [2002] *PARIHS* model; and Rogers's [2003] *Diffusion of Innovations* theory) of implementation or translation science to investigate adoption of research-based practices (Nilsen, 2015; Titler, 2010). There are also formal programs of *knowledge-translation research* aimed at evaluating strategies to change nurses' behaviors (e.g., Wallin, 2009)

TABLE 6.1 Patterns of Knowing and Evidence for Practice and DNP Projects

Pattern of Knowing	Description	Evidence for Practice
Empirics	Factual, descriptive, publicly verifiable, generalizable May be context specific	Randomized controlled trials; original research. Translating findings to practice settings through quality improvement innovations
Aesthetics	The art of nursing. Gaining knowledge of another person's experience through empathetic acquaintance	Reflective practice along the novice-to-expert continuum
Personal knowing	Knowing, encountering, and actualizing self	Therapeutic use of self in patient engagement
Ethics	Moral choices regarding voluntary actions within specific contexts	Developing own philosophy of nursing. Aligning own beliefs with standards of practice

Source: Carper (1978).

and *logic models* as devices for planning, implementation, and evaluation (see Urban & Trochim, 2009, for a review). Existing work in this area continues to evolve.

DNP projects may take many forms, from pilot studies for practice change initiatives and basic descriptive studies that examine relationships among key factors to program evaluation, quality improvement (QI) projects, and testing new practice models. DNP projects often involve QI. QI is a process by which individuals work together to improve systems and processes of care delivery with the intention to improve outcomes (Newhouse et al., 2011). The aim of QI is to improve operational activities and the connections within, working toward the goal of safe, timely, and efficient patient-centered care (S. J. Brown, 2014). The linking theme across these forms of inquiry is the use and translation of systematically obtained empirically informed evidence to improve practice or patient outcomes.

CLINICAL SCHOLARSHIP: A DUAL PROCESS

Autonomy of practice depends on nursing having a scientific body of knowledge for practice. Autonomy of practice mandates that advanced practice nurses provide care at the highest level and that they have additional expertise in the development, implementation, and evaluation processes that generate knowledge to improve practice. Clinical scholarship is an intellectual process of inquiry that not only *implements* interventions but challenges interventions, tests, and ideas, predicts outcomes, and explains patterns and exceptions through observation, analysis, synthesis, application, and dissemination (National Organization of Nurse Practitioner Faculties [NONPF], 2016).

Nurses engage in a wide variety of research methods, including and perhaps especially those that fit the study of problems relevant to specific contexts of nursing practice. And the scope of nursing theories, which has moved down the ladder of abstraction from grand to middle level and situation-specific theories, can facilitate the DNP research project with its particular focus on practice.

Figure 6.1 depicts the interrelationships among the nursing metaparadigm, the four domains of knowledge, theoretical models, evidence-based practice, and the DNP project. The overarching metaparadigm organizes broad conceptual focuses of nursing. The metaparadigm is represented through selected nursing and nursing-related theories that inform evidence-based practice and guide the DNP project. Relationships among the elements in the figure are very fluid in that knowledge embedded in each can influence other domains in a way supportive of the nonlinear process of knowledge translation between research and practice. In addition to research-based evidence, the interacting elements that inform knowledge translation include various stakeholders, patient and family values and health experiences,

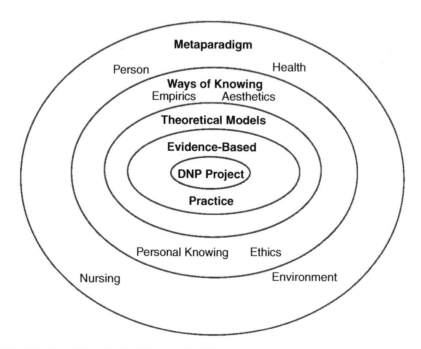

FIGURE 6.1 Relationship among theory, evidence-based practice, and DNP project.

contextual and cost factors, as well as the nurse's own clinical expertise and ethical and personal patterns of knowing.

Thus, the DNP student is an evolving clinical scholar as one who "uses evidence-based practice skills to translate current best evidence to improve health care and health care outcomes, thereby transforming systems of care" (NONPF, 2016, p. 1). Through dual processes of research and practice, the DNP graduate will be able to effectively translate knowledge of research into practice. Each of these processes is represented in a model for knowledge translation taught to DNP students, described in the following section.

MODELS TO GUIDE THE DNP PROJECT PROCESS

KNOWLEDGE TO ACTION FRAMEWORK

One approach that is fitting for DNP students and DNP-prepared advanced practice nurses is the *Knowledge to Action Framework* (Straus, Tetroe, & Graham, 2009). A particular advantage of this model, unlike other knowledge translation models, is that its framework incorporates the research process and the practice dimension, both of which are vital in the knowledge translation of clinical scholarship. The ongoing and complex interactions between the creation and production and use of knowledge facilitate the innovative process of translating knowledge for practice. What is important to note is that it is through processes inherent in both scientific *research* and evidence-based *practice*, knowledge is generated, critiqued, refined, and translated for practice.

Knowledge creation consists of *three phases*:

1. Knowledge inquiry
2. Synthesis
3. Tools and products of knowledge creation

These phases are cyclical, since knowledge creation is not static but undergoes critique and refinement to become more useful to the end users of the knowledge, such as researchers, health care providers, and policy makers.

Knowledge application involves *seven action phases*:

1. Identifying the problem
2. Reviewing and selecting the knowledge to implement

3. Adapting or customizing the knowledge to the local context

4. Assessing knowledge use determinants

5. Selecting, tailoring, implementing, and monitoring knowledge translation interventions

6. Evaluating outcomes or impact of using the knowledge

7. Determining strategies for ensuring sustained knowledge use

These action phases can occur simultaneously with the three knowledge creation phases, and interactions between phases influence action phases at several points in the cycle. Action parts are based on planned action theories that focus on practice change within health care systems and groups.

Key to the process is the consideration of the end user/stakeholders and foreseeing expected outcomes (Straus et al., 2009, p. 7). Often DNP students create third-generation knowledge, for example, clinical practice guidelines, decision aids, and educational modules, which are one end product of knowledge development within the context of their projects.

PROJECT PROCESS MODEL

The *Project Process Model* developed by Zaccagnini and White (2017) highlights the key steps in the DNP project development and is congruent with the action phases of the *Knowledge to Action Framework*. Developed by two DNP-prepared advanced practice registered nurses, this model was one of the first specific to the DNP project and includes *nine steps*:

1. Problem recognition

2. Needs assessment

3. Goals, objectives, and mission statement

4. Theoretical underpinnings

5. Work planning

6. Evaluation planning

7. Implementation

8. Interpretation of data

9. Utilization and reporting of results (p. 450)

Overall, the basic steps of the scientific method provide the foundation for any QI project. Other frameworks appropriate for DNP QI projects, depending on their purposes, are the Institute for Health Improvement's Model for Improvement (MFI; Langley, Moen, Nolan, Norman, & Provost, 2009), Lean (IHI, 2005; Konig, Verver, van den Heuvel, Bisgaard, & Does, 2006), and Six Sigma (Konig et al., 2006). Lean was developed by Toyota and other Japanese companies as an integrated system of principles, practices, tools, and techniques designed to reduce waste and manage workflows (Konig et al., 2006). Six Sigma originated by Motorola with emphasis on decision making based on analysis of data and focused on cost reduction measures (Konig et al., 2006). The most common model used for DNP projects is the MFI, by which three questions are posited: (a) What are you trying to accomplish? (b) How will you know that a change is an improvement? and (c) What change can be made that will result in an improvement? Sources for various models on the DNP project development processes are presented in several texts (Bonnel & Smith, 2014; Moran, Burson, & Conrad, 2017; Zaccagnini & White, 2017).

SQUIRE GUIDELINES

An additional resource to augment models that guide the DNP project research process is the *SQUIRE* (Standards for Quality Improvement Reporting Excellence) guidelines (Ogrinc et al., 2015). These guidelines provide a framework for reporting on QI projects, and in doing this they also provide a structure that students may use in developing their DNP project. The SQUIRE guidelines were initially published in 2008 following a consensus among health care leaders and academicians who wanted to consolidate the evidence for a science of improvement. The guidelines, with a subsequent checklist, have been used to systematically and objectively develop and evaluate scholarly publications related to health care improvement. In 2015, SQUIRE 2 was published following several revisions. This edition is designed to apply across methods such as iterative changes in single settings, which is a common scenario for DNP students (Ogrinc et al., 2015).

The SQUIRE guidelines provide a template for reporting research findings regarding practice knowledge and changes that improve health care and health outcomes. This template can be adapted for DNP projects to incorporate specific items related to advanced practice nursing and recommendations from the AACN. The general questions in the template align with steps in other models used to guide the DNP project.

The following four questions are presented in the guidelines and can assist students in preparing a formal document, such as their final document for the graduate college or for a publication of their DNP project.

1. *Why did you start this QI project?*
   This question helps the student think through how the clinical problem was determined, the nature and significance of the local problem, and relevant supporting data. By this, the student shapes the statement of the purpose of the project and the study question to be answered. The nature and significance of the local problem to incorporate relevant data and available knowledge are included. This section can be tailored to advanced practice nursing by adding

the significance to health care and advanced practice nursing. The *purpose of the study* with a practice-related study question is supported through a synthesis of evidence about what is currently known about the problem. Concepts, *theoretical frameworks*, or *models* are used to explain the problem and to guide the development of the project's procedure, approach, or intervention.

2. *What did you do?*
   In answering this question, the student describes the method of the study. The DNP project is often context specific and often occurs within one practice setting. Therefore, a clear and full description of the setting and the population is important. Ethical aspects must be addressed to ensure protection of human subjects. The project design must correlate with the purpose and problem statement. A description of the study procedure, any interventions, and data collection methods and measurement tools for studying the processes and outcomes is provided. Enough detail of the methods is provided to facilitate replication of the study in another setting. The rationale for selecting a certain design, intervention, and measures selected for studying the processes and their outcomes are also explained. Data analysis is also described, and may include both quantitative and qualitative methods.

3. *What did you find?*
   In addition to addressing the results, this section also demonstrates the DNP student's ability to reflect and find meaning from the project process and results providing detail of the process measures and outcomes within the context of the practice. The complexity of practice-based research is often evident given its "real-world" practice setting and the unintended consequences that often occur related to benefits, costs, collaboration, communication, and other contextual factors.

4. *What does this mean?*
   Perhaps the most important section for demonstrating the synthesis of student learning in the DNP project process is the final section, discussing the results. Through the lens of the advanced practice nursing student and evolving clinical scholar, several areas are addressed: (a) the link from the results back to the theoretical framework of the study; (b) the link between the current results and extant evidence—whether they support previous results from research; (c) implications of the findings for advanced nursing practice and health care specific to a population, including their link to existing practices; and (d) last, if a practice change is indicated by the results, how will its sustainability be ensured?

The final step of any DNP project is dissemination of the practice knowledge generated by the DNP project. The results are reported through several venues, most importantly with key stakeholders. Dissemination to health care professionals also facilitates transferability of the results to similar practice settings.

THE FUTURE OF DNP CLINICAL SCHOLARSHIP

A distinguishing feature of the DNP graduate's expertise and role is clinical scholarship that integrates the various sources of knowledge from advanced nursing practice and practice-informed research to generate transferable research findings. DNP students' academic preparation is founded on advanced practice principles, experiential learning, collaboration, and application of current evidence-based practices. Their academic preparation also involves acquiring tools for developing scientific knowledge, such as designs for QI and program evaluation, and methods of analysis and synthesis. These and other skills and knowledge facilitate development of nurses who can support translation of knowledge for quality health care.

Just as human health and health care are complex processes, DNP projects will be diverse in the questions they address, in the theoretical perspectives for framing the focus and interpreting the findings, and in their designs, methods, implementation processes, and evaluation. As the DNP movement, grounded in practice, evolves, it is likely that new perspectives and innovations will emerge as well. These will advance thinking about linkages between research and practice, theory-based practice models, and the transfer and transformation of knowledge that occur through the dual processes of nursing practice and scientific inquiry.

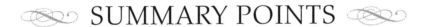 SUMMARY POINTS

1. The DNP project is a mechanism for teaching the generation and translation of nursing practice knowledge to stimulate research and improve clinical outcomes.

2. Knowledge translation involves the nurse's use of many patterns of knowing—research and practice-based, ethical and personal.

3. Several models are available to guide the DNP project process and dissemination.

4. The integration of practice-based research and practice-based evidence is a dual process that contributes to clinical scholarship for enhancing patient outcomes and health care system change.

QUESTIONS FOR REFLECTION

1. How would you describe "translating research into practice" to a colleague?

2. What are characteristics of a DNP project that enable generation of practice-relevant knowledge?

3. What resources does a practitioner have that facilitate translation of research findings into practice?

4. What are strengths of the various models presented in the chapter?

 REFERENCES

Agency for Healthcare Research & Quality. (2001). Fact sheet: Translating research into practice (TRIP)-II. AHRQ Pub. No. 01-P017. Retrieved from https://archive.ahrq .gov/research/findings/factsheets/translating/tripfac/trip2fac.html

American Association of Colleges of Nursing. (2006). *The essentials of doctoral education for advanced practice nursing.* Washington, DC: Author.

American Association of Colleges of Nursing. (2015). *The doctor of nursing practice: Current issues and clarifying recommendations: Report from the task force on the implementation of the DNP.* Washington, DC: Author. Retrieved from http://www.aacn .nche.edu

Auerbach, D. I., Martsolf, G., Pearson, M. L., Taylor, E. A., Zaydman, M., Muchow, A., . . . Dower, C. (2014). *The DNP by 2015-A study of the institutional, political, and professional issues that facilitate or impede establishing a post-baccalaureate doctor of nursing practice program.* RAND Corporation. Retrieved from https://www.ncbi.nlm.nih.gov/pmc/ articles/PMC5158236

Bonnel, W., & Smith, K. V. (2014). *Proposal writing for nursing capstones and clinical projects.* New York, NY: Springer Publishing.

Brown, M. A., & Crabtree, K. (2013). The development of practice scholarship in DNP programs: A paradigm shift. *Journal of Professional Nursing, 29*(6), 330–337.

Brown, S. J. (2014). *Evidence-based nursing: The research-practice connection* (3rd ed.). Burlington, MA: Jones & Bartlett.

Carper, B. A. (1978). Fundamental patterns of knowing in nursing. *Advances in Nursing Science, 1*(1), 3.

Dols, J. D., Hernández, C., & Miles, H. (2017). The DNP project: Quandaries for nursing scholars. *Nursing Outlook, 65*(1), 84–93.

Institution for Healthcare Improvement. (2005). *Going lean in health care*. IHI innovation series white paper. Cambridge, MA: Author.

Kitson, A., & Harvey, G. (2016). Methods to succeed in effective knowledge translation in clinical practice. *Journal of Nursing Scholarship, 48*(3), 294–302.

Kitson, A., Harvey, G., & McCormack, B. (1998). Enabling the implementation of evidence based practice: A conceptual framework. *Quality in Health Care, 7,* 149–158.

Konig, H., Verver, J., van den Heuvel, J., Bisgaard, S., & Does, R. (2006). Lean Six Sigma in healthcare. *Journal for Healthcare Quality, 28*(2), 4–11.

Langley, G. L., Moen, R., Nolan, T. W., Norman, C. L., & Provost, L. P. (2009). *The improvement guide: A practical approach to enhancing organizational performance* (2nd ed.). San Francisco, CA: Jossey-Bass.

McArthur, D. B. (2017). The journey to the doctor of nursing practice degree. In K. Moran, R. Burson, & D. Conrad (Eds.), *The doctor of nursing practice scholarly project—A framework for success* (2nd ed., pp. 15–34). Burlington, MA: Jones & Bartlett.

Moran, K., Burson, R., & Conrad, D. (Eds.). (2017). *The doctor of nursing practice scholarly project—A framework for success* (2nd ed.). Burlington, MA: Jones & Bartlett.

National Organization of Nurse Practitioner Faculties. (2016). White paper: The doctor of nursing practice nurse practitioner clinical scholar. Retrieved from http://c.ymcdn.com/sites/www.nonpf.org/resource/resmgr/docs/ClinicalScholarFINAL2016.pdf

Newhouse, R. P., Stanik-Hutt, J., White, K. M., Johantgen, M., Bass, E. B., Zangaro, G., . . . Weiner, J. P. (2011). Advanced practice nurse outcomes 1990–2008: A systematic review. *Nursing Economic$, 29*(5), 230–250.

Nilsen, P. (2015). Making sense of implementation theories, models and frameworks *Implementation Science, 10,* 1–13.

Ogrinc, G., Davies, L., Goodman, D., Batalden, P., Davidoff, F., & Stevens, D. (2015). SQUIRE 2.0 (Standards for QUality Improvement Reporting Excellence): Revised publication guidelines from a detailed consensus process. *British Medical Journal Quality & Safety, 25*(12), 986–992. doi:10.1136/bmjqs-2015-004411

Rogers, E. M. (2003). *Diffusion of innovations* (5th ed.). New York, NY: The Free Press.

Rycroft-Malone, J., Kitson, A., Harvey, G., McCormack, B., Seers, K., Titchen, A., & Estabrooks, C. A. (2002). Ingredients for change: Revisiting a conceptual framework. *Quality and Safety in Health Care, 11,* 174–180.

Straus, S., Tetroe, J., & Graham, I. D. (2009). *Knowledge translation in health care—Moving from evidence to practice*. West Sussex, United Kingdom: Blackwell.

Titler, M. G. (2010). Translation science and context. *Research and Theory for Nursing Practice: An International Journal, 24*(1), 35–55.

Urban, J. B., & Trochim, W. (2009). The role of evaluation in research-practice integration: Working toward the "golden spike." *American Journal of Evaluation, 30*(4), 538–553.

Wallin, L. (2009). Knowledge translation and implementation research in nursing. *International Journal of Nursing Studies, 46,* 576–587.

Zaccagnini, M. E., & White, K. W. (Eds.). (2017). *The doctor of nursing practice essentials-A new model for advanced practice nursing* (3rd ed.). Burlington, MA: Jones & Bartlett.

Interlude II: *Mindfulness and Knowledge Development in Nursing Practice*

Catherine Johnson

Nursing knowledge generation in the 21st century is radically changing from the research and theory development activities of the past. With the advent of the first universally acknowledged practice doctorate in nursing degree (the doctor of nursing practice [DNP]) and changing perspectives of evidence beyond that espoused by positivist philosophy, nursing practice experts are poised to become significant participants in knowledge development. The contemplative practice of mindfulness is an approach that not only enhances patient care but also can open a space to expand attentive awareness of oneself and the situation to facilitate knowledge development in the context of nursing practice.

The emergence of contemplative practice is coming at a time in the history of science that has increasingly found evidence of a broader definition of phenomena, beyond that which can be explained by mechanistic processes. Nursing science has a foundation in empirical scientific methods but is rapidly expanding to describe and explicate nursing phenomena through alternative ways of knowing, including the qualitative approaches of ethnography and phenomenology. Awareness, attention, and concentration are critical skills for researchers observing and describing the nature of phenomena. Nurturing awareness, attention, and concentration is at the heart of mindfulness and can strengthen research efforts and knowledge development. The contemplative practice of mindfulness on a simple process, such as breathing, can be a useful means of strengthening awareness, attention, and concentration. I invite you to explore the ideas presented here on mindfulness practice in reference to your own work in nursing.

Because of the constantly changing practice environment, research findings and extant theories can become outdated, perhaps quickly becoming no more than historical information about a point in time (Jarvis, 2000). However, mindfulness practice as a reflective practice may enhance the knowledge we already obtain from extant research and theories when it is applied to the changing practice context. Expert nurses can increase their attention to their experiences in practice and unlock their own practice knowledge. Mindfulness practice can increase understanding of clinical patterns and their meanings—as grounded in the expert nurses' mindful awareness of their own beliefs and values, assessments and decisions, and knowledge and experiences. Reflective practice is often described as a window through which previously unseen dynamics and implications for knowledge within the nurse–patient interaction can be revealed (Trelfa, 2005).

MINDFULNESS AND EXPANDED AWARENESS

Over the past decade, mindfulness has garnered increased attention and supporting evidence across a variety of health-related disciplines (Christopher & Maris, 2010). Jon Kabat-Zinn (1994), a pioneer of mindfulness practice, defined *mindfulness* as "paying attention in a particular way, on purpose, in the moment and non-judgmentally" (p. 4). Mindfulness practice also has been described as "open, undivided observation of what is occurring both internally and externally rather than a particular cognitive approach to external stimuli" (Brown & Ryan, 2003, p. 823). The mindful practitioner attends to his or her sensory and cognitive processes in a nonjudgmental way during everyday tasks to aid clarity and insight regarding their everyday reality. A strength of the mindful practitioner is an expanded capacity to maintain emotional balance within any particular life moment. To practice mindfulness is to cultivate awareness of being alive in the present moment (Solloway & Fisher, 2007). Deepening this awareness leads to being more present and experiencing life more vividly, yet also being aware of life's impermanent nature. *Mindfulness*, then, refers to an expanded awareness characterized by a purposeful and nonjudgmental attending to the present moment.

Paying attention is the prime objective of mindfulness. Through this process of discovery, practitioners can observe their own experiences while participating in them. The correct attitude toward this process can be summarized by the words of Gunaratana (2002):

> *Never mind what I have been taught. Forget about theories and prejudgments and stereotypes . . . I want to understand the true nature of life. I want to know what this experience of being alive really is. I want to apprehend the true and deepest qualities of life, and I don't want to just accept somebody else's explanation. I want to see it for myself.* (p. 18)

The foundational attitudes of mindful practice have been defined by Jon Kabat-Zinn (1994) and Thich Nhat Hanh (1998) as:

1. *Non-judging:* taking the stance that you are an impartial witness of your own experience

2. *Patience:* letting things unfold in their own time

3. *Beginner's mind:* cultivating a mind that is willing to see everything as if for the first time

4. *Trust:* trusting in yourself, your feeling, and your own authority and intuition

5. *Nonstriving:* paying attention to how you are right now—however that is

6. *Acceptance:* seeing things as they actually are in the present

7. *Letting go:* letting go is a way of letting things be, of accepting things as they are

All cultures in the world have a history of some mental practice designed to assist people in living and coping with the stresses of their world through increased understanding. These practices vary greatly, but overall they include the elements of conscious thought, concentration, and reflection (Gunaratana, 2002). Within the Buddhist tradition, not only is concentration highly valued but equally so is the element of awareness that occurs with mindfulness. As part of the Noble Eightfold Path, mindfulness is at the heart of Buddha's teachings. Mindfulness is said to be the energy that can bring about understanding and insight through careful attention and concentration (Hanh, 1998).

INSIGHT MEDITATION

Vipassana, or insight meditation, is the oldest Buddhist meditation practice and involves the gradual cultivation of mindfulness or awareness. Some evidence suggests that Vipassana may be useful clinically although more research is indicated (Chiesa, 2010). With insight meditation, the meditator's attention is focused on certain aspects of her or his own experience through observation of the flow of life experiences moment to moment. Insight meditation is a mindfulness practice that focuses on breathing while sitting in a meditative state. There are mindfulness practices that involve other physical activities, which also aid in bringing mindfulness into everyday life. These include walking meditation or yoga postures. All are focused on developing awareness of "being in the body, with a mind" (Moss & Barnes, 2008, p. 12).

THE CHALLENGE OF CONCENTRATION

Insight meditation fosters development of mindfulness in part by increasing the ability for concentration. Concentration is regarded as a key tool in achieving enhanced awareness or mindfulness. Through this ancient form of sensitivity training, insight meditation helps a person become more receptive to life experiences by attentively listening, observing, and testing the reality experienced in the moment without judgment or bias. The enhanced concentration developed through meditation can become a natural approach to reflecting on your inner and external experiences in mindfulness practice.

The process of focusing on the realm of thoughts and the present moment is a daunting one. The mind is incredibly active, and if your focus is on paying attention to your senses, thoughts, and feelings in any given moment, you will soon be overwhelmed.

The concentration is not about being mindful of something in particular; to be mindful *of* something separates self from the present reality. Instead, the concentration has more to do with being mindful *in* the present. As Muho Noelke (2004) stated in a lecture he gave while he was the Abbott at Antaiji, a Zen monastery:

> . . . *We have to forget things like "I should be mindful of this or that." If you are mindful, you are already creating a separation. . . . Don't be mindful, please! When you walk, just walk. Let the walk walk. Let the talk talk. . . . Let the eating eat, the sitting sit, the work work. Let sleep sleep.* (para. 2)

For this reason, in the early stages of the meditative process, a focus on a concrete entity is especially helpful in maintaining concentration. As mentioned, a common entity used in insight meditation is the breath because breathing is a part of everyone's experience. This concentration on the breath in meditation is a tool to move you into the realm of the present moment and to achieve and sustain present-focused awareness or mindfulness.

RESEARCH ON MINDFULNESS

The increasing impact of mindfulness and its relevance to nursing practice is evident through a review of articles and research studies in nursing on mindfulness published over the 5-year time frame of 2011 to 2015. A total of 211 articles were found, focusing on clinical practice areas, educational settings, and leadership and professional development applications. This broad application of mindfulness to these prominent domains of nursing may signal the utility of mindfulness and reflective practice as a facilitator of improved leadership and clinical outcomes and knowledge development within nursing. The following articles highlight key findings from this pool of published works and demonstrate sophistication in their conceptualization and applications of mindfulness as well as their evaluation of mindfulness as an intervention.

A concept analysis of mindfulness in nursing using Rodgers's evolutionary method of concept analysis was completed by White (2014) in which 59 articles from 1981 to 2012 were reviewed. Data were analyzed focusing on attributes, antecedents, consequences, references, and related terms in relationship to mindfulness in the nursing literature. Five attributes of mindfulness were identified: the experience of *being present;* three attributes that sustain *being present: awareness, acceptance, and attention;* and mindfulness as a *transformative process* for participants. Antecedents to the practice of mindfulness include the desire to commit, time to practice, patience, and persistence. The consequences of mindfulness for nurses and their patients are well documented, including stress reduction and lower levels of depression and pain. This study found that mindfulness is a significant concept within nursing. The author did point out that applications of mindfulness in nursing education, practice, and leadership have increased, yet research activity and methods lag behind. The majority of the research studies reviewed were quantitative and many demonstrated insufficient statistical power. Improved research methods, including the increased use of qualitative methods, were recommended in order to adequately evaluate the outcomes of mindfulness and its contribution to nursing science and practice.

Hunter (2016) expanded understanding of the impact of mindfulness on practicing nurses and midwives through the critical interpretative synthesis of five articles found in CINAHL, Medline, and PsycINFO databases that met all inclusion criteria. The author identified themes in this review and developed a "mindfulness cascade." This depiction of the impact of mindfulness training on nurses and midwives included five distinct processes that empowered the nurses and midwives and resulted in improved patient care. These processes are

1. *Gaining control:* putting aside negative thoughts and *controlling* brain chatter, leading to calm and peace, resulting in increased self-efficacy.

2. *Time and space:* gain *agency* over actions and develop new *perspectives* of self and their place in their environment.

3. *Improved care:* increasing attention and awareness of patients' and colleagues' needs.

These depictions are consistent with other findings on the positive impact of increased mindfulness among health care providers.

Ponte and Koppel (2015) described the implementation of the mindfulness-based stress reduction program developed by Jon Kabat-Zinn with nursing clinical staff in a large cancer treatment center. Components of this program included training in mindful meditation, mindful movement (yoga, tai chi), and body scan. Sixty staff members participated, and through postintervention surveys the authors found that participants identified increasing productivity, decreased stress, and increased feelings of control and accomplishment, resulting in increased ability to be available to their patients and attend to their needs.

Anderson and Guthery (2015) evaluated the impact of a mindfulness psychoeducational program for parents of children with attention-deficit/hyperactivity disorder (ADHD). This 8-week program used the text *Everyday Blessings: The Inner Work of Mindful Parenting* by Myla and Jon Kabat-Zinn.

Their postintervention evaluation of parental stress, using the Parenting Stress Index, fourth edition, Short Form (PSI-4-SF), found a significant reduction in parental stress consistent with the findings of Bogels, Hellemans, van Deursen, Romer, and van der Meulen (2014).

Pipe, FitzPatrick, Doucette, Cotton, and Arnow (2016) presented findings from their action learning team project as part of the Robert Wood Johnson Foundation Executive Nurse Fellowship. Five video interviews were presented that provided real-life examples of how nurses employ mindfulness in their clinical and leadership practice. The aim of this project was to increase understanding of the power of mindfulness in nursing practice. The authors found that participants felt they were better able to objectively observe automatic and habitual behaviors as well as their own coping patterns and thought processes. By paying attention with focus and purpose through mindfulness they were better able to focus on the present and be more effective leaders and clinicians.

Increasing use of mindfulness in higher education has been stimulated through the works of Arthur Zajonc. Building on the work of the philosophers Goethe and Steiner, Zajonc has developed the field of contemplative inquiry, which bridges the gap between traditional scientific beliefs and research with the emerging field of contemplative inquiry. As a professor of physics at Amherst and director of academic programs of the Center for Contemplative Mind in Society, Zajonc has focused on a new framework for transformational education. This contemplative pedagogy and its methods are described as educating the whole person by integrating the inner and outer life in order to achieve a broader understanding and compassion for themselves, others, and society (Palmer, Zajonc, Scribner, & Nepo, 2010). This new approach acknowledges the increasing community of scholars who seek new ways of knowing that link the objective with the subjective and the analytic with the integrative.

Nursing has been a leader in mindfulness in education. Increasingly, methods including reflective learning through blogs and journaling, mindful exercises, and meditation are used by undergraduate and graduate faculty. These approaches to mindfulness practice are of interest because they may facilitate new as well as expert nurses' abilities to see new concepts and make connections that might otherwise be missed in the clinical situation. The positive impact of meditation and mindfulness on learning and perceiving may have implications in helping nurses become cognizant of their personal theories and develop concepts relevant to their clinical practice.

Research by Solloway and Fisher (2007) into the measurement and effects of mindfulness practice generated results that may have implications for developing nursing knowledge in practice. Their study involved 338 undergraduate students and a comparison over time and across two groups, those who received mindfulness training and those who did not receive the training. Methodological results indicated that mindfulness is "teachable, learnable and amenable to measurement" (Solloway & Fisher, 2007, p. 69). Substantive findings suggested that mindfulness training in novice practitioners affects an increase in "psychological strengths," including increased emotional balance, being a more attentive listener, feeling more positive about accomplished tasks, noticing things in nature never noticed previously, increased insight, and increased ability to examine life without being caught up in the process (Solloway & Fisher, 2007, pp. 70–71).

These effects of mindfulness practice are of interest because they may facilitate nurses' abilities to see new concepts and make connections that might otherwise be missed in the clinical situation. The positive impact of meditation and mindfulness on learning and perceiving may have implications for helping nurses become cognizant of their personal theories and develop concepts relevant to their clinical practice.

OUTCOMES OF MINDFULNESS IN NURSING PRACTICE

In mindfulness practice, one becomes aware of the present moment and every thought and feeling as an inner monologue emerges. Mindfulness practice creates an attentive, intelligent quality in each element of one's experience, yet does not focus on "figuring it out"; rather, the mindful nurse merely observes these parts of experience in a nonjudgmental way. The capacity of simply being aware and accepting the present moment is the desired outcome of mindfulness practice. Openness to the flow of thought and increased attention to the present moment occur as one practices mindfulness. Unexpected outcomes, fears, or desires are acknowledged but are not dwelled upon as one increases appreciation of the quiet wisdom within.

An important outcome of mindfulness is the development of compassion, a critical element of caring. Mindfulness has been described as a purification of the mind, particularly in reference to ego processes of greed and hatred. Transformational exercises are often used to prepare the meditator with a mantra of "universal loving kindness" (Gunaratana, 2002). This exercise includes speaking the following intention before meditation practice and repeating it in full, focusing on your "self" and then on your teachers, relatives, friends, and enemies, and last on all living beings:

> *May I live well, happy and peaceful. May no harm come to me. May no difficulties come to me. May no problems come to me. May I always meet with success.*
>
> *May my teachers live well, happy and peaceful. May no harm come to them. May no difficulties come to them. May no problems come to them. May they always meet with success. . . .* [and so on in reference to others.]. (Gunaratana, 2002, p. 4)

These universal loving kindness intentions are meant to guide you as the meditator in transformation of your speech and actions toward yourself and all living beings and to prepare you for meditation and mindfulness practice.

Insight meditation facilitates development of mindfulness. However, mindfulness is not contained in the meditative process only. Mindfulness can be cultivated in the context of everyday life through gentle reminders to maintain awareness of whatever is happening moment to moment. Mindfulness provides a clearer perspective of both self and the present situation.

There are both personal and professional benefits to be gained by engaging in this meditative process. Within your personal life, you may experience increased calm and satisfaction in the world around you when you focus on the quiet contemplation of meditation and on the universal loving kindness intentions. In the professional realm, you may find yourself more available to your patients, interacting with them in a calm, compassionate manner. You may also find that you are more available to your team members and be able to support them more compassionately and consistently.

POTENTIAL KNOWLEDGE-BASED OUTCOMES

Mindfulness practice is a strategy to enrich nursing practice and increase opportunities for nurses to develop theoretical ideas derived from their professional practice experiences. Mindfulness can facilitate knowledge development in nursing practice through awareness and integration of various ways of knowing in nursing, such as that involved in the personal theories Rolfe (1998) suggested are developed by expert nurses in practice.

Developing personal theory in practice must involve personal knowledge—that is, awareness of your philosophy of nursing and beliefs about practice—and all nurses possess a philosophy whether or not they have articulated it. Trelfa (2005) advised that reflective practice cannot be divorced from the professional's beliefs and feelings but is linked to one's worldview and practice philosophy. Avis and Freshwater (2006) urge careful examination of practitioners' beliefs and thought processes, all viewed as influences in their interpretation of evidence and the resultant decisions made in practice. In addition, the Buddhist practice of insight meditation as it supports mindfulness practice can help nurses break down these complex thought processes through expanded awareness of their sensory and cognitive experiences.

New mental habits can be attained through the ongoing practice of meditation and subsequent ability to deal with conscious thought and sensory experiences. When practicing mindful, nonjudgmental awareness of your surroundings and nursing actions, you as the nurse may see areas for enhancing your own professional development as well as for improving the effectiveness of patients' own health care strategies. Professional health care providers, then, are challenged to use mindfulness practice to explore and articulate emotional and cognitive elements of their practice and then revisit these definitions in light of new self-awareness. The following scenario is an example of how mindfulness practice helped the author gain awareness of the emotional and theoretical elements embedded in a challenging clinical situation.

EXAMPLE OF MINDFULNESS PRACTICE IN A CONTEXT OF VIOLENCE

The process of mindfulness may parallel processes that practicing nurses have already experienced. Expert nurses often may see beyond the nursing theories that they have been taught to perceive their clinical situations *in the moment* as a natural flow of the elements they seek to understand. In what is often described as an intuitive process, they see the *whole* and react to the situation in a comprehensive way. This perception is very similar to mindfulness in that expert nurses break away from the previously described experiences of others and trust their own perceptions and insights. In doing this, they identify and link together pertinent concepts, building their own theories to explain what is occurring in the present moment. Practicing nurses' personal theories evolve out of heightened awareness of this moment and the simultaneous integration of knowledge about the underlying process taking place.

I experienced this awareness in my practice as a family nurse practitioner in Deming, New Mexico. I had been practicing mindfulness meditation for some time and was becoming increasingly aware of moment-to-moment experiences that I felt as energy flowing around me. Several incidents of violence had occurred both in our clinic and in the small community of Deming. I, along with the clinic staff, felt anxious and unsafe.

As I became increasingly mindful through daily meditation, I began to feel less anxiety and more comfortable and at peace. I also experienced an increase in my non-judgmental awareness of the situation, which resulted in an increase in my effectiveness as a team member and practitioner. My acceptance of the situation and my awareness of my own anxiety and that of the other staff members helped me talk more freely with my teammates about these feelings and how they might have an impact on our patients. We as a team were then able to look at our clients as part of the same environment we were experiencing and its influence on all of us. As I became more a part of the present experienced by my clients, I could purposefully include this shared awareness in my assessments, decisions, and plans. I increased my ability to provide compassionate care by being in the present moment with myself, my teammates, and my clients. Together, we joined in the present and became more at peace, supported, and effective.

My mindfulness practice involved a reflecting-*in*-practice that increased my awareness and understanding of the situation and enhanced my actions with clients and my team. Next, as a second step in using mindfulness to develop nursing knowledge, I reflected on this scenario, a kind of reflection-*on*-practice, to further explicate and refine what began as my personal theory that emerged in the situation. Here is my stream of theoretical ideas from my personal theory:

- Mindfulness practice helped me reflect on a problematic situation and gain increased awareness of my own anxiety.

- Increased awareness facilitated my open discussion of concerns among the team.

- This open discussion, in turn, helped the team and me perceive clients as part of the same environment and as having similar anxieties and fears.

- This perception enabled me to purposefully share my perceptions with clients and obtain a fuller assessment of their concerns in the process.

- This perception also enhanced my compassion toward clients and my ability to convey this to clients.

- Expanded knowledge of the situation coupled with my compassionate approach in my nursing practice led to more effective interventions and better teamwork in the clinic.

NEXT STEPS

A next step in building nursing knowledge is to connect existing theory and research and other practitioners' experiences with my personal theory. I would use these sources to support or challenge the string of inferences I drew from my clinical observations and reflections and to identify key concepts that may be linked together to organize a theoretical framework. The framework would propose an explanation of what was happening in that clinical situation. This framework would be generated from a synthesis of all the available evidence. It would then be tested through research methods and by practicing nurses who share a similar concern with enhancing health care provider well-being, teamwork, and client care in the context of threats of violence.

Thus, through the practice of mindfulness, nurses can achieve greater understanding of their environment and their practice, specifically through the tools of concentration and heightened awareness of self and the clinical situation. Mindfulness practice not only increases the number of elements that nurses factor into their clinical strategies and actions but also widens the opportunities for identifying new concepts that may better explain clinical phenomena. Mindfulness practice enables the nurse to take a crucial mental step away from the clinical situation to perceive all of the elements involved in a situation and in the actions taken and to evaluate clinical dynamics and outcomes. This understanding not only contributes to our practice wisdom but also provides an opportunity for concept and theory development.

A STEP-BY-STEP GUIDE FOR INSIGHT MEDITATION LEADING TO MINDFULNESS

The following is a step-by-step guide to participating in insight meditation (Gunaratana, 2002). Meditation is an experience that is learned through experience and practice. Guidance through this process by a knowledgeable teacher is required for greatest success.

1. Dress in loose soft clothing that will not restrict circulation. No belts or thick material. Shoes and socks or stockings should be taken off.

2. Traditional Asian postures are sitting on the floor with a cushion to elevate the spine. A chair can be used, however. Focus of posture is to choose one that allows you to remain immobile without pain for the entire length of the meditation.

3. Determine how long you are going to meditate based on how long you can sit immobile without pain. Beginners should start with not more than 20 minutes of meditation. Time is not the focus for success; progress is.

4. After positioning yourself and sitting motionless, close your eyes.

5. Share your universal loving kindness intentions.

6. Take three deep breaths, then breathe normally, letting your breath flow in and out freely. Focus your attention on the *rim of your nostrils*. Simply notice the *feeling of breath* going in and out. These are the *first two objects* of focus for meditation.

7. Ignore any thought, memory, sound, smell, or taste. Focus exclusively on the breath.

8. As you continue, you will notice that initially the inhalation and exhalation are short and rapid, but with increased awareness you will notice them becoming longer as your mind and body become calm.

9. As you continue, you will begin to notice that the entire breathing process becomes more subtle. A calm and peaceful feeling of breathing will come.

10. Despite your best efforts, your mind may wander and you may be focused on your friends, your family, bills you need to pay, and so on. As soon as you notice you are no longer focused on your breath, return to a focus on the rim of your nostrils and your inhalation and exhalation. Counting can be used to assist you in staying focused. For example, you can count 1–1–1–1 with the next inhalation and 2–2–2–2 with the next exhalation. Continue up to five cycles counting up to 10. Repeat as needed until your breathing is quiet and barely noticed.

11. As the breath gets more quiet and subtle, your mind and body can feel so light it feels like you are floating. You will begin to be aware of an *image or sensation,* which is a sign of meditation and is the *third object* of meditation. This may appear as a star, the moon, a long string, or film of clouds. It is unique to you and it means you have reached the state of concentration sufficient for insight meditation and mindfulness.

12. At the end of the meditation session (indicated by the sound of a bell in some settings), you will slowly open your eyes and be aware of the environment. You will feel calm and peaceful. Move carefully and quietly because this is a transition period that must be taken slowly.

With consistent and patient practice, you can develop deepening levels of concentration that will increase your ability to develop mindfulness. This building process may take months to years, and for most meditators, it is a lifelong quest. However, soon after initiating the meditation practice, you can experience results by an increase in peacefulness and calm (Gunaratana, 2002).

MINDFULNESS AND THE FUTURE OF SCHOLARLY PRACTICE

Mindfulness is a strategy that can enrich nursing practice and increase opportunities for nurses to develop theoretical ideas out of their professional practice. Increased use of mindfulness as a nursing intervention that focuses on increasing awareness, attention, and self-efficacy for patients in a variety of settings has been well described and evaluated in recent nursing publications. Similarly, Sigma Theta Tau

International (Freshwater, Horton-Deutsch, Sherwood, & Taylor, 2005) promotes meditation and mindfulness practice as a strategy to enhance reflective practice, proposed as an overall means to "encourage deeper levels of analysis and interpretation of nursing issues relating to practice" (p. 3). The practice of insight meditation and the development of expanded awareness, attention, and concentration through mindfulness practice enable nurses to examine their thoughts, decisions, knowledge base, and feelings and reflect on the entire process within a patient–nurse interaction.

Mindfulness, as a process similar to Schön's (1983) reflection-in-action, can increase nurses' capacities to attend to patients' needs and enhance practice knowledge in their constantly changing practice environments (Freshwater et al., 2005). From this new level of awareness *in* practice as well as from later reflections *on* practice, nurses can evaluate and refine their own knowledge base and improve clinical practice.

Research is needed to better understand the potential for mindfulness to promote scholarly practice, specifically the impact of mindfulness on the nurse's awareness and use of personal theories to extend concept and theory development in nursing. Mindfulness has the potential to provide both the individual nurse and the profession a means to better understand the complex practice environment of nursing care and the reality of nursing practice within this environment. Exploration of mindfulness as a knowledge-enhancing process may provide critical insights into the practice wisdom of expert nurses, as nursing expands its practice boundaries with the practice doctorate and seeks to identify and measure the unique contributions of this new role in nursing.

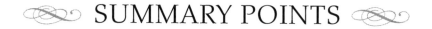

SUMMARY POINTS

1. As a contemplative practice, mindfulness can be a useful strategy to enrich nursing practice and increase opportunities for nurses to develop theoretical ideas out of their professional practice.

2. Mindful nurses may experience increased awareness, attention, and focus that support the development of deeper understanding of their nursing practice and the complex environment within which they are practiced.

3. Better understanding of the dynamics of mindfulness and its outcomes will assist in expanding its usefulness as a practice intervention, professional development, and educational strategy, as well as theory development opportunity.

4. Expanded research and reflective practice approaches are needed to expand and promote scholarly practice, specifically the impact of mindfulness on the nurse's awareness, attention, and focus and the use of personal theories to extend concept and theory development in nursing.

QUESTIONS FOR REFLECTION

1. Reflecting on the mindfulness practice example, what theoretical ideas might you identify?

2. What nursing experiences have you had in which mindfulness practice might be useful in promoting your own or clients' well-being?

3. The chapter outlined a guide for insight meditation leading to mindfulness practice that can be followed by DNP and PhD nurses. How might you use insight meditation in your own practice to move nursing knowledge forward in a new way?

4. What are some of the challenges you might face when engaging in mindfulness practice to provide patient care and build knowledge?

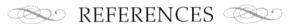 REFERENCES

Anderson, S., & Guthery, A. (2015). Mindfulness-based psychoeducation for parents of children with attention-deficit/hyperactivity disorder: An applied clinical project. *Journal of Child and Adolescent Psychiatric Nursing, 28*, 43–49.

Avis, M., & Freshwater, D. (2006). Evidence for practice, epistemology and critical reflection. *Nursing Philosophy, 7*, 216–224.

Bogels, S., Hellemans, J., van Deursen, S., Romer, M., & van der Meulen, R. (2014). Mindful parenting in mental health care: Effects on parental and child psychopathology, parental stress, parenting, coparenting, and marital functioning. *Mindfulness, 5*, 536–551.

Brown, K. W., & Ryan, R. M. (2003). The benefits of being present: Mindfulness and its role in psychological well-being. *Journal of Personality and Social Psychology, 84*, 822–848.

Chiesa, A. (2010). Vipassana meditation: Systematic review of current evidence. *Journal of Alternative and Complementary Medicine, 16*(1), 37–46.

Christopher, J. C., & Maris, J. A. (2010). Integrating mindfulness as self-care into counseling and psychotherapy training. *Counseling and Psychotherapy Research, 10*(2), 114–125.

Freshwater, D., Horton-Deutsch, S., Sherwood, G., & Taylor, B. (2005). *Position paper on the scholarship of reflective practice*. Indianapolis, IN: Sigma Theta Tau International. Retrieved from https://www.nursingsociety.org/docs/default-source/position-papers/resource_reflective.pdf?sfvrsn=4

Gunaratana, H. (2002). *Mindfulness in plain English*. Somerville, MA: Wisdom.

Hanh, T. N. (1998). *The heart of the Buddha's teachings.* New York, NY: Broadway Books.

Hunter, L. (2016). Making time and space: The impact of mindfulness training on nursing and midwifery practice: A critical interpretative synthesis. *Journal of Clinical Nursing, 25,* 918–929.

Jarvis, P. (2000). The practitioner-researcher in nursing. *Nurse Education Today, 20,* 30–35.

Kabat-Zinn, J. (1994). *Wherever you go there you are: Mindful meditation in everyday life.* New York, NY: Hyperion.

Moss, D., & Barnes, R. (2008). Birdsong and footprints: Tangibility and intangibility in a mindfulness research project. *Reflective Practice, 9*(1), 11–12.

Noelke, M. (2004, October). Adult practice 18: Stop being mindful. *Lotus in the fire.* Shin'onsen, Japan: Antaiji. Retrieved from http://antaiji.org/archives/eng/adult18.shtml

Palmer, P., Zajonc, A., Scribner, M., & Nepo, M. (2010). *The heart of higher education: A call to renewal.* Hoboken, NJ: Wiley.

Pipe, T., FitzPatrick, K., Doucette, J. N., Cotton, A., & Arnow, D. (2016). The mindful nurse leader: Improving processes and outcomes: Restoring joy in nursing. *Nursing Management, 47*(9), 44–48.

Ponte, P., & Koppel, P. (2015). Cultivating mindfulness to enhance nursing practice. *American Journal of Nursing, 115*(6), 48–55.

Rolfe, G. (1998). *Expanding nursing knowledge: Understanding and researching your own practice.* Oxford, United Kingdom: Butterworth Heinemann.

Schön, D. A. (1983). *The reflective practitioner: How professionals think in action.* New York, NY: Basic Books.

Solloway, S., & Fisher, W. (2007). Mindfulness in measurement: Reconsidering the measureable in mindfulness practice. *International Journal of Transpersonal Studies, 26,* 58–81.

Trelfa, J. (2005). Faith in reflective practice. *Reflective Practice, 6,* 205–212.

White, L. (2014). Mindfulness in nursing: An evolutionary concept analysis. *Journal of Advanced Nursing, 70*(2), 282–294.

8

Creating a Nursing Intervention out of a Passion for Theory and Practice

Nelma B. Crawford Shearer

There is considerable literature on how to develop nursing interventions. Some instruct that nursing interventions are developed from a systematic review of literature to link the identified problem or phenomena of concern with research efforts (Polit & Hungler, 1995). Others emphasize theory as driving the development of intervention (e.g., Sidani & Braden, 1998; Whittemore & Grey, 2002). My focus is to discuss an extension of approaches to developing theory-based intervention, emphasizing the role of clinical practice. This practice-oriented approach is an iterative process in which practice enriches theory and serves as a guide to creating a theory-based intervention. This chapter chronicles programmatic research in developing a theory-based nursing intervention designed to foster health empowerment. The main purpose is to encourage nurses to develop their own ideas from clinical practice into theory-based intervention.

Developing a theory-based intervention is not a linear process. It is an iterative process of working back and forth between practice experiences and theoretical perspectives while keeping an eye on the research findings regarding the practice problem. Learning about the nature and characteristics of theory and theory development strategies during PhD coursework gave me some of the tools needed to imagine an intervention. Theory came alive as I reflected on my own philosophy or worldview (beliefs and values) about nursing and nursing practice. A course in middle-range theory guided me through a variety of nursing theories and in merging theory with practice experiences to frame an intervention using theoretical concepts from my own perspective. From these foundational courses, I developed, tested, and continued to refine the health empowerment theory using qualitative and quantitative research methods.

REFLECTING ON PRACTICE EXPERIENCES

Nursing practice provides a foundation for knowledge production (Reed, 2006). Reflection on experiences in clinical and community health practice during PhD study provided a basis for clarifying philosophical worldview, identification and analysis of core concepts for theory development, testing, and refinement.

Practice Example 1: During my undergraduate clinical practice experience in community health, I visited a woman on her family farm. The woman had been in a car accident and suffered a fracture to her hip. She was able to move around her home with the use of crutches but was not able to stand on her feet for a long time. While completing the assessment, it became apparent that what was bothering her most was the need to organize her kitchen to prepare family meals. This meant rearranging her kitchen cupboards and moving items to within-chair-level reach. I stopped and asked myself: *Should I rearrange her kitchen to make it more manageable; would this be perceived as a nursing role?* I did rearrange the woman's kitchen, and, in retrospect, I enacted a tacit nursing theory about health that helped this woman live according to what was meaningful and healthy to her in the context of her health concerns. For this woman, health was defined as being able to prepare meals for her family; for me, nursing was defined as facilitating her ability to purposefully participate in attaining this meaningful goal. This encounter links to my current theory of practice, the enactment of which empowers individuals to participate knowingly in change and in so doing provides knowledge for nurses to directly intervene in the situation.

Practice Example 2: After graduation, I worked in a rural hospital to polish my technical skills. One afternoon, I began making rounds and encountered an older female patient who was crying. As I tried to comfort her, she told me a story about her daughter and how she had drowned in a flash flood. Despite the fact that I should have been passing afternoon medications to a variety of patients, I took the time to sit with her, listen to her story, and stayed with her until she stopped crying. When I got ready to leave, she graciously thanked me for listening and told me that sharing her daughter's story made her feel better. She commented that she knew I had more important things to do for other patients. Reflecting on this experience later during my doctoral studies, I realized that listening and providing support as well as helping individuals find ways to help themselves were components of my emerging theory of health empowerment.

Practice Example 3: Through my teaching experiences in a large metropolitan clinic, I often witnessed nurses creating a standardized plan of care for the sick children rather than working with the mother to create a personalized care plan specific to her children. The mothers were not always able to follow through with the standardized plan of care and returned to the clinic because the children's health had not improved. Nurses often grumbled about the returning mothers' failure to follow the plan of care and labeled them *frequent fliers* and noncompliant. In fact, the nurses appeared puzzled when the mothers consistently failed to adhere to the prescribed plan of care for their children. Reflecting back and guided by my theory of practice, the mothers should not have been prescribed standardized care plans. Instead, their children should have been given individualized plans based on nurse and mother working together and on the child's needs.

CLARIFYING MY PHILOSOPHIC WORLDVIEW

An initial step in theory development involved formulating a philosophic worldview of nursing science consistent with values, beliefs, and practice experiences. Articulating a worldview included views of human beings, their health, and practice as a "useful process in knowledge development" (Reed, 2011, p. 8). In particular, reading and discussion about the contextual-dialectic worldview from Pepper (1948), life-span developmental literature (Lerner, 1997), Parse's (1987) simultaneity and Newman's (1992) unitary-transformative worldviews from nursing, and Rogers's Science of Unitary Human Beings (Rogers, 1970, 1980, 1990, 1992) helped clarify my philosophic views. The *contextual-dialectic worldview* focuses on the dynamic relationship between human beings and their environment; human beings are continuously changing and growing in the midst of conflict. *Life-span development* is an ongoing historical event that has the potential for qualitative as well as quantitative change. The *simultaneity paradigm* presents human beings as synergistic with the environment, with health as individually defined. The *unitary-transformative worldview* focuses on human beings as integral with their environment, identified by pattern rather than biopsychosocial parts, and changing in ways that are not deterministic, that is, change cannot be controlled or predicted. Human beings and the environment from the perspective of Rogers's (1992) Science of Unitary Human Beings are unitary, irreducible, indivisible, pandimensional energy fields in mutual process. In other words, because a person and environment function as one unit, their influences on each other are continuous, complex, and never completely predictable.

Key assumptions underlying my worldview included (a) observations about phenomena must include focus on the individual as well as on the person's interaction with the environment; (b) health is an approach to life; and (c) definitions of health differ with each human being (Shearer 2000, p. 20).

CONCEPT ANALYSIS AND CLARIFICATION

The concept of *empowerment* captured my interest and influenced my philosophical view of nursing. Consistent with the assumptions underlying my worldview, in practice I had witnessed women who experienced frustration when prescribed standardized care rather than receiving a personalized care plan that reflected their definition of health and access to resources. I was of the opinion that the women should have been listened to, supported, and encouraged to actively participate in developing their treatment plans.

To better understand the concept of empowerment I conducted a concept analysis, exploring the use, assumptions, and disciplinary perspectives in use of the concept. The concept analysis and clarification involved two phases, both of which, it is important to note, were influenced by my worldview. For example, the literature review focused on health rather than illness, with a view of human beings as active participants in their health and health care.

The *first phase* followed Walker and Avant's (2005) guidelines in which the attributes, antecedents, and outcomes associated with empowerment were identified from a synthesis of research and theory literature. The attributes of empowerment reflected a belief in self, personal strengths and abilities, choice, control over factors affecting one's life, recognition, transformation, resources, and a desire or willingness to take action as participation in change.

In the *second phase,* I formulated statements of association and conditional relationships between empowerment and related concepts as a beginning step in theory development (Walker & Avant, 2005). In the relationship statements, I proposed that empowerment was positively associated with personal control, high self-esteem, autonomy, health, and well-being, as well as levels of control over life, consciousness, participation, and relationship. Conditional statements identified empowerment as linked to people and resources and a sense of personal competence with willingness to take action.

The concept analysis uncovered two very different assumptions: Some authors viewed empowerment as an inherent developmental process, whereby empowerment included levels or steps, with a person becoming increasingly empowered. Others viewed empowerment as a social process in which empowerment occurred as a result of external forces acting on a person and affecting the person's sense of control and feeling of power (Shearer & Reed, 2004).

DEFINITION OF EMPOWERMENT

As a result of the concept analysis and statement clarification, I defined empowerment as an inherent developmental process, *facilitating a transforming belief in self.* Framing empowerment as a developmental process captured the role of individuals' perceptions and definitions of health in their mutual process with the environment, while choice and a transforming belief in self reflected health as individually defined and a positive approach to life.

RESEARCH

INITIAL QUALITATIVE WORK

Building on the findings of the concept analysis, I conducted qualitative research using *phenomenological* methodology to discover the meaning of the lived experience of health empowerment among women with children. I focused on women because I regarded women as gatekeepers of their families' health and believed that empowered women could better care for themselves as well as their families. The use of a qualitative approach allowed me to incorporate my practice experiences, worldview, and concept analysis to better explain the nuances and dimensions of health empowerment in the words of women themselves.

For women, the lived experience of health empowerment often began with a health event, whereby their own values and goals conflicted with approaches to care proposed by health care providers. For example, one woman was overprescribed pain medication for chronic back pain, with no attention to relevant lifestyle changes such as physical activity, weight loss, or relaxation. Realizing that the pain medication was impacting her roles as a mother and wife, not to mention her personal needs, she began to explore other approaches to managing her pain, taking control of her health in ways that corresponded to her personal values and reflected her own patterns of health. The women shared "aha" moments of recognizing that they had a choice to knowingly participate in what they chose for themselves in behaviors consistent with their own health patterns, fostering belief in themselves and their own judgment.

This transforming belief in self, enacting valued choices, and knowing participation in their health behaviors were fostered through nurturing and encouraging self-talk that affirmed their strengths. The presence of supportive others as social support reinforced a sense of personal choice in health care decisions. Consistent with my philosophic worldview and concept analysis, health empowerment emerged as a transforming belief in self through self-talk and support from others (a person–environment mutual process) and to participate knowingly in their own health and health care (health patterning), reflecting health as an individually defined and positive approach to life (well-being).

QUANTITATIVE WORK

The initial qualitative research provided the foundation for research designed to *develop and test a theoretical framework or model of health empowerment in women* (Shearer, 2004). I proposed a developing framework of health empowerment for quantitative evaluation of the relationships between theoretical constructs (Figure 8.1). The construct *person–environment* was defined as an evolving, ever-changing unitary (or mutual) process of human beings and environment, as based on Rogers's (1992) principle of integrality depicting human beings as integral with their environments in their daily livings and health experiences. *Person–environment* was conceptualized as reflecting: (a) **contextual factors** (operationalized as personal profile characteristics including age, income, years of education, number of children, and number of years married) and (b) **relational factors** (operationalized as social support and professional support). The construct *health-patterning* was defined as a dynamic process of engaging women to participate knowingly in change. Health empowerment, as an indicator of health patterning, was defined as "the transforming belief in one's ability to participate knowingly in health and health care decisions" (Shearer, 2000, p. 31) manifesting itself in health behavior and awareness of choices to participate knowingly in change (operationalized as knowing participation in change and as health behaviors).

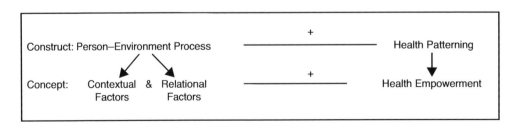

FIGURE 8.1 Theoretical model.

The framework was tested in a sample of 123 women with children, aged 21 to 45. Results provided partial support for my theoretical idea that empowerment emerges from both person and environmental factors—the person–environment mutual process. A higher level of education and social support (representing environmental factors) and the person's *knowing participation in change* were all important in explaining health empowerment (Shearer, 2004). There was still need, however, to further examine the explanatory ability of contextual and relational factors, and my next activities provided this opportunity.

At this juncture in my research and practice career, I became involved with the older adult population through my community health practice and experiences with my own aging parents (Shearer, 2002). These experiences informed my research. I recognized that older adults may view health empowerment differently from other groups including middle-aged and younger women. Thus, I returned to qualitative research to better understand the contextual and relational factors explaining health empowerment among community-dwelling older women.

ADDITIONAL QUALITATIVE WORK

The results from two additional qualitative studies provided further support for my theory in proposing key factors that facilitate health empowerment. A study with focus groups of community-dwelling older women (Shearer & Fleury, 2006) provided detailed descriptions of social-contextual resources (encouragement, information, nurturance, and feedback in negotiating life changes in aging). Results from a phenomenological study (Shearer, 2007) supported the theory and also provided insights from the lived experiences of homebound older women that helped explain how *social-contextual resources* and *personal resources* facilitated health empowerment. Social contacts and supportive networks enhanced the women's ability to stay connected and remain in their own homes. And more importantly, *personal resources,* in terms of women's inherent capacity for change and growth, facilitate health empowerment. These findings provided direction for the focus on my nursing intervention.

Revising My Theory

I used the findings from the qualitative studies to revise and refine the health empowerment theoretical framework to include *personal resources* (initially called contextual factors) and *social-contextual resources* (initially called relational factors). I arrived at a view of health empowerment as a relational process emerging from the woman's *recognition* of personal resources and social-contextual resources (Shearer, 2007). Through the health empowerment process, a transformation occurred in the woman's awareness of and belief in her ability to participate knowingly in the changes inherent of health and health outcomes. This view involved a shift from a paternalistic perspective in which the health care provider establishes the goals to one where the homebound older woman participates knowingly in determining and

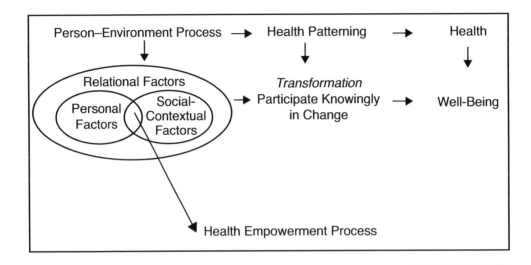

FIGURE 8.2 Theoretical framework.

progressing toward attainment of personal health goals, thus promoting well-being (Figure 8.2).

QUANTITATIVE WORK—INTERVENTION STUDY

I constructed the *Health Empowerment Intervention* (HEI) as guided by my health empowerment theory (Shearer, 2000, 2004, 2009). The problem to be addressed by the intervention was discovered from my practice and research experiences. I found that women, particularly homebound older women, were at risk for losing their independence as their health needs became more complex; and their ability to achieve valued health goals seemed to be limited because they were unaware of resources. To enhance a homebound woman's health empowerment, I proposed that she first had to become aware of her resources, specifically *personal resources* and *social-contextual resources*. Figure 8.3 depicts the HEI framework, the variables, and their relationships within the health empowerment theoretical framework and the intervention mechanisms (Shearer, Fleury, & Belyea, 2010).

TRANSLATING THE HEI
TO PRACTICE

From a practice perspective, the focus of the HEI was to address the homebound older woman's personally relevant health goals and means to attain these goals. The nurse

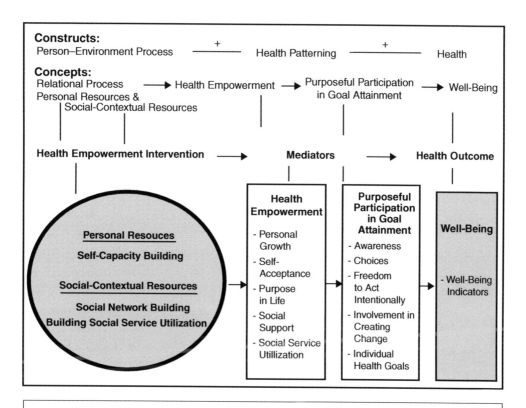

FIGURE 8.3 Health empowerment intervention framework.

in concert with the woman facilitates engagement in the process of recognizing personal resources, including self-capacity, and social-contextual resources, including social network and access to social services. In addition, the HEI addressed personally relevant health goals and concerns for each homebound older woman and the means to attain these goals (Shearer, 2009).

Practice encounters that are guided by the theory of health empowerment and the HEI involve facilitating health on the women's terms and in the context of the moment (Shearer, Fleury, & Reed, 2009). A nurse practicing from a health empowerment perspective promotes the woman's awareness of and engagement in personal and social-contextual resources first and foremost by listening to her (Practice Example 2). Nursing actions are then directed at helping an older woman become aware of and use resources to purposefully participate in working toward the attainment of health goals (Practice Examples 1, 2, and 3). Thus, the nurse in concert with the older woman engages in a participatory process in which the nurse listens and encourages the older adult to talk, share, and enact her health goals (Shearer, 2009).

In practice, the nurse would focus on helping the woman recall and/or build awareness of *personal resources* through constructive reminiscence of a time when the woman felt able to overcome a challenge. Reminiscence can be thought of as memory release in which life experiences are poured out and used to facilitate self-capacity building through the acknowledgment of strengths. One strategy a nurse would use to increase awareness of *social-contextual resources* is facilitating problem-solving methods to help the woman identify persons and community resources that supported her in the past. Building on this recognition, the woman then accesses and engages new resources to attain her health care goals. In addition, role-playing facilitates reconnecting with others, seeking needed help, and contacting and communicating with social service agencies to access needed resources (Shearer, 2009).

THE INTEGRALITY OF MY RESEARCH, PRACTICE, AND THEORY-BASED INTERVENTION

The theory-based HEI involved an iterative process where practice and research findings enriched my theorizing and served as a guide in creating the intervention. Explicating my theory-based intervention did not occur overnight, nor was it guided by a single design or research method. Results from use of diverse research methods along with reflection on clinical practice experiences were integrated into my evolving theory, to develop and refine the intervention. It was important to clarify my philosophic views and beliefs as a basis for theory development and refinement, given my passion for promoting well-being in vulnerable populations and for understanding—from a nursing perspective—the human health experience.

In this ongoing program of research, I continue to explore person and environmental factors that facilitate health empowerment and positive health outcomes (Shearer et al., 2010; Thakur, Fleury, Shearer & Belyea, 2017). Given my dual passions for practice and theory, it is gratifying that my research goals lead to new ways of linking practice with theory and to discovering how theory can enrich practice. New thinking in this direction will help promote an awareness of the full spectrum of factors that may optimize health of older adults.

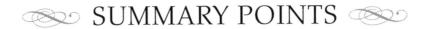 SUMMARY POINTS

1. Clinical practice is offered as a perspective in the development of theory-based intervention.

2. Developing a theory-based intervention is an iterative process that incorporates practice experiences along with theoretical perspectives and research findings.

3. Explicating a theory-based intervention does not occur overnight, nor is it guided by a single design or research method.

QUESTIONS FOR REFLECTION

1. What practice experiences have left their footprints in your mind?

2. What are you passionate about in nursing? Is it theory, practice, research, or a combination?

3. How do you see yourself becoming a scholar and creator of a theory-based intervention?

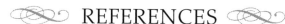 REFERENCES

Lerner, R. (1997). *Concepts and theories of human development* (2nd ed.). Mahwah, NJ: Lawrence Erlbaum.

Newman, M. A. (1992). Prevailing paradigms in nursing. *Nursing Outlook, 40,* 10–13, 32.

Parse, R. (1987). Paradigms and theories. In R. Parse (Ed.), *Nursing science: Major paradigms, theories, and critiques* (pp. 1–11). Philadelphia, PA: Saunders.

Pepper, S. P. (1948). *World hypotheses: A study in evidence.* Berkeley: University of California Press.

Polit, D. F., & Hungler, B. P. (1995). *Nursing research: Principles and methods* (5th ed.). Philadelphia, PA: Lippincott Williams & Wilkins.

Reed, P. G. (2006). The practice turn in nursing epistemology. *Nursing Science Quarterly, 19*(1), 51–60.

Reed, P. G. (2011). The spiral path of nursing knowledge. In P. G. Reed & N. B. C. Shearer (Eds.), *Nursing knowledge and theory innovation advancing the science of practice* (pp. 1–35). New York, NY: Springer Publishing.

Rogers, M. E. (1970). *An introduction to the theoretical basis of nursing.* Philadelphia, PA: F. A. Davis.

Rogers, M. E. (1980). A science of unitary man. In J. P. Riehl & C. Roy (Eds.), *Conceptual models for nursing practice* (2nd ed., pp. 329–337). New York, NY: Appleton-Century-Crofts.

Rogers, M. E. (1990). Nursing: Science of unitary, irreducible, human beings: Updated 1990. In E. Barrett (Ed.), *Visions of Rogers' science-based nursing* (pp. 5–11). New York, NY: National League for Nursing.

Rogers, M. E. (1992). Nursing science and space age. *Nursing Science Quarterly, 5,* 27–34.

Shearer, N. B. C. (2000). Facilitators of health empowerment in women (AAT 9965911; Doctoral dissertation, University of Arizona, 2000). *Dissertation Abstracts International, 861*(3), 1–144.

Shearer, N. B. C. (2002). Loss of power within the nursing home zone. *Journal of Gerontological Nursing, 28*(1), 54–56.

Shearer, N. B. C. (2004). Relationships of contextual and relational factors to health empowerment in women. *Research and Theory for Nursing Practice, 18,* 357–370.

Shearer, N. B. C. (2007). Toward a nursing theory of health empowerment in homebound older women. *Journal of Gerontological Nursing, 33*(12), 38–45.

Shearer, N. B. C. (2009). Health empowerment theory as a guide for practice. *Geriatric Nursing, 30*(2, Suppl. 1), 4–10.

Shearer, N. B. C., & Fleury, J. (2006). Social support promoting health in older women. *Journal of Women & Aging, 18*(4), 3–17.

Shearer, N. B. C., Fleury, J., & Belyea, M. (2010). Randomized control trial of the health empowerment intervention. *Nursing Research, 59,* 203–211.

Shearer, N. B. C., Fleury, J., & Reed, P. G. (2009). The rhythm of health in older women with chronic illness. *Research and Theory for Nursing Practice, 23,* 148–160.

Shearer, N. B. C., & Reed, P. G. (2004). Empowerment: Reformulation of a non-Rogerian concept. *Nursing Science Quarterly, 17,* 253–259.

Sidani, S., & Braden, C. S. J. (1998). *Evaluating nursing interventions: A theory-driven approach.* Thousand Oaks, CA: Sage.

Thakur, R., Fleury, J., Shearer, N. B. C., & Belyea, M. (2017). *Optimizing self-management in older adults with heart failure—A feasibility study.* Unpublished paper presented at the Western Institute of Nursing 50th Annual Communicating Nursing Research, Denver, CO.

Walker, L. O., & Avant, K. C. (2005). *Strategies for theory construction in nursing* (4th ed.). Upper Saddle, NJ: Pearson/Prentice Hall.

Whittemore, R., & Grey, M. (2002). The systematic development of nursing interventions. *Journal of Nursing Scholarship, 34*(2), 115–120.

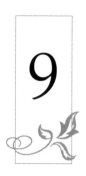

9

Interlude III: *Practitioner as Theorist: A Nurse's Toolkit for Theoretical Thinking in Nursing*[1]

Pamela G. Reed

Inquiry is

a natural activity that is as intimately related to organic nature as the beating of a heart and the perches and flight of a bird. . . . It arises from felt needs, employs both abstract and concrete tools, tests proposals in the laboratory of experience, and terminates in the resolution of the difficulties which occasioned that particular sequence of inquiry. (Hickman, 2007, p. 37)

Thomas Kuhn's (1962/1970) *The Structure of Scientific Revolutions* exploded into a controversy about scientific inquiry that continues into this century (Fuller, 2000). We know from writings of science historians, sociologists, and philosophers that the practice of science changes over time. Perspectives and strategies of knowledge development change as well. Nearly 50 years ago, nursing scholar Rosemary Ellis (1969) published her idea of the *practitioner as theorist*, which today marks a new path of knowledge theory development that can expand our repertoire of strategies for knowledge production in nursing. Nursing practitioners are an untapped resource

1. Adapted from P. G. Reed (2008). Practitioner as theorist: A reprise. *Nursing Science Quarterly,* *21,* 315–321. Reprinted by permission of Sage Publications.

for generating nursing theories to guide research and practice that enhance human well-being and health care.

MAKING PRACTITIONERS' THEORIZING EXPLICIT

The ability to theorize is a fundamental characteristic of human beings, the foundation of which is developed early in life and extends to the intentional activities of scientists (Ellis, 1969; Kaplan, 1964; Magnani, 2001; Vosniadou, 2001). Writings revealing the integrality of theory and practice and the potential for theory development among practitioners have increased over the past two decades. For example, Fawcett and colleagues (Fawcett, Watson, Neuman, Walker, & Fitzpatrick, 2001) expanded the field of theorizing with their application of Carper's (1978) pluralistic paradigm of nursing knowledge. Doane and Varcoe (2005) fused theory and practice together in their concept of *compassionate action*. And Chinn's (Chinn & Kramer, 2015) *praxis*, first discussed decades prior to this edition, denoted the transformative process of developing knowledge through critical practice.

Theories and theorizing are embedded in practice, as many scholars have attested. An important next step is to address Ellis's (1969) original appeal to nursing to make practitioners' theorizing explicit. In her words,

> If we really have a commitment to the future beyond the personal accumulation of wisdom from patient to patient, and if we wish to communicate this wisdom we must . . . have practitioners in nursing who are willing to be scholars as well and who have the interest, skill, and time to pursue the analyses and formulations [of nursing theories] and test them in practice. (p. 1438)

Advancements in models of the nursing process have helped make more explicit the thinking strategies used in practice. However, these models typically focus on decision making, problem solving, critical thinking, or diagnostic and clinical reasoning. They do not focus on developing theory-based knowledge in practice—neither in terms of a methodology of theory development nor in terms of a substantive base of knowledge about human health processes. As Ellis (1969) pointed out, nurses may categorize assessment data, identify patterns, and form concepts, but they often stop short of advancing a theory by identifying links between concepts and outcomes of nursing care.

HISTORICAL TRENDS IN THEORY DEVELOPMENT

Nursing has a history of theory-development activities that have generated a diverse and dynamic structure of knowledge. Theoretical systems range from broad philosophic and paradigmatic statements, to conceptual models, middle-range theories, and theories that focus on specific practice situations. Approaches to developing nursing knowledge in the context of practice have changed over time and reflect changes in philosophies of science.

NIGHTINGALE AND EMPIRICISM

Florence Nightingale's 19th-century approach to theory development was influenced by British empiricism, which upheld the primacy of the five main senses in scientific knowledge. Her theorizing took the form of empirical generalizations, presented as canons in her *Notes on Nursing* (Nightingale, 1859/1969). Nightingale worked horizontally on the empirical plane, using analogic reasoning to generalize across observations of patients and their environment, and then to organize specific statements about nursing and health. For example, from her observations of air, water, drainage, cleanliness, and light, she generalized statements about the *health of houses* and wrote a special section on that in her book.

Nightingale's theoretical statements were relational but not explanatory. She could *describe* a situation well and with her statistics predicted outcomes and reduced mortality rates. However, she did not have the conceptual tools to address health phenomena by explaining *how* or *why* environmental factors such as noise from the chattering hopes of visitors and music or the colors in varieties of flowers affected patient mood. That required theorizing vertically up to more abstract levels to access unseen (and therefore unaccepted) mystical concepts, such as sound and light waves, and psychological phenomena to explain a patient's well-being.

PEPLAU AND POSTPOSITIVISM

Peplau's mid-20th-century approach to theorizing reflected postpositivist views dominant at the time, along with a dramatic shift from Nightingale's emphasis on *nursing as doing* to a focus on *nursing as knowing*. Peplau's theorizing allowed for abstract concepts and she applied her knowledge of interpersonal theories and underlying mechanisms, such as the psychodynamics of behavior and therapeutic milieu, to explain the healing power of nursing therapy. Her practice methodology centered on the nurse–patient relationship within a therapeutic environment. This was her context of knowledge production.

The corpus of Peplau's writings (e.g., Peplau, 1988) presents a method of knowledge development that shifts between nursing practice and formal research. Peplau's *cycle of inquiry* (Reed, 1996) begins in the context of the nurse–patient relationship. The nurses' observations become the fundamental theoretical units, which are spiraled up drawing in relevant theories. Theoretical explanations are then *peeled out* from what the nurse has observed. The resulting theory is applied, tested, and transformed into nursing knowledge in the crucible of nursing practice.

ROGERS AND INTERMODERNISM

Theorizing in the 21st century reflects shifts in philosophy away from modernism toward postmodernism and post-postmodernism (or intermodernism [Reed, 2011]) in which theories are no longer regarded as stable ideas that correspond to a higher truth but more as conceptual systems of ideas that influence and are influenced by their context. Although postmodernism decentered positivist and foundationalist notions of theory, theory nonetheless is still valorized as a prestigious activity across disciplines (Chaiklin, 2004).

Intermodern (Reed, 2011; formerly called neomodern in Reed, 2006; Whall & Hicks, 2002) views reflected in theory development include the following: pluralism in sources of knowledge and methods of theory development; pragmatism balanced by assumptions about the mystery of life; belief in the capacity of human beings for innovation, agency, and well-being; an openness to change and critique; and valuing local truths as well as broader philosophies for their perspectives on what is emancipating, good, and healthful and other goals in nursing practice.

Rogerian thought (Rogers, 1970) is evident in the participatory and holistic perspectives underlying 21st-century nursing theorizing. Parse's (1987) *simultaneity* paradigm provides for nursing a discipline-defining alternative discourse to the medical model of health care: one that privileges patient perspectives and participation and values the nurse caregiver in knowledge production. Newman's *unitary-transformative* (UT) worldview (Newman, Sime, & Corcoran-Perry, 1991) identified substantive focuses for theory development such as the person's inherent potential for self-organization, innovative patterning, and connection to the environment. Cowling (2007) operationalizes Rogerian philosophy in his description of participatory action research, which united researchers, if not practitioners, and patients in the quest for nursing knowledge.

TOWARD PARTICIPATORY METHODS: AREAS FOR DIALOGUE

Theory building that includes the patient as partner (as well as the practicing nurse) equalizes the power between patients and nurses and fosters partnerships rather than paternalism in knowledge endeavors. The aim, as Barker (1999) warns in his discussion of nursing aspirations for professional status, is not *"to develop a professional, expert, and esoteric body of knowledge to be kept from, yet applied to the 'patient,'"* ... [this is] *"antithetical to the idea of partnership and reciprocity identified as the way forward in health care"* (p. 68).

It is time to reconsider assumptions about how knowledge development may occur and evaluate whether current methods align with our philosophies about nursing and science. There is need for dialogue and study on theory-development strategies that have fit and relevance in practice.

Questions for dialogue include the following:

- What traditional methods could be modified or reformulated as well as what new methods can be devised to better facilitate practitioner and patient involvement in knowledge development?
- What kind of participation do patients and families desire?
- What are the ethical considerations of practice-based theory development?
- Are practitioners interested in participating more actively in developing nursing knowledge?
- Do nurses care, as Peplau did, to *know* the why and how behind what they *do*?
- What resources are needed to do this in the practice setting?
- How can educational curricula support the learning needs of practitioners as knowledge producers?

EXTANT METHODS AND TOOLS FOR THEORY INNOVATION

In addition to the standard nursing theory textbooks that address theory development strategies, there are methods and tools of clinical inquiry that are potentially useful to practitioners in generating theory. These include grounded theory methodology, clinical reasoning, structured reflection, participatory action research, and clinical conceptual frameworks. *Grounded theory methodology* is flexible and can be adapted to practice situations (Glaser, 1978; J. Holton for B. Glaser, personal communication, June 6, 2008). It is a method grounded in patient caregiving processes, which include assessment and observation, organizing and interpreting data, identifying links and patterns in the data, and validating findings with the patient. A comprehensive work in *clinical reasoning* by Kuiper, O'Donnell, Pesut, and Turrise (2017) extends scholarly work on critical thinking to study dimensions of clinical reasoning that may become tools for practice-based theory development. Rolfe and Gardner's (2005) *reflexive model of evidence-based practice* combines strategies of action research and Schön's (1983) reflection-in-action and single-case experimentation to form and test hypotheses relevant to nursing care in a specific patient care situation. Reed and Lawrence (2008) described structures called *clinical conceptual frameworks* as a mechanism for clinicians to transform interactions with patients and other data into theory form. The frameworks can be used to help clinicians articulate and formalize their personal theories and identify areas of inquiry in patient care.

NEW PERSPECTIVES

Less conventional tools and strategies for theorizing may evolve out of the dynamic context of nursing practice. New perspectives on theory development may be helpful in stimulating thinking on how to facilitate practice-based theory development and, as Ellis (1969) pleaded, make practitioner theories more explicit.

GUERRILLA THEORIZING

Guerrilla theorizing describes one perspective on how nurses in practice may engage in theory development. This concept, derived in part from the dynamic nature of nursing practice coupled with intermodern views from nursing and contemporary science, emphasizes participatory practices, the person–environment process of change, pragmatism and pluralism in knowledge building, and voices of patients and bedside caregivers in nursing theory and practice. The etymology of the term *guerrilla* indicates that the word means *small war*, the diminutive of the Spanish term for war, *Guerra*. The word originated in the early 1800s in reference to the Spanish resistance against Napoleon (*Webster's New Universal Unabridged Dictionary*, 1996). However, the term has come to have wide application as an adjective to describe strategies not of warfare but of bold and creative human endeavors ranging from *guerilla puzzling* as a model for scientific research to guerilla art, photography, marketing, graphic design, and even garage sales and an online physician group fighting back against the corporatization of health care.

Guerrilla-based strategies are unconventional, culturally sensitive, embedded or integrated in the local context, and dedicated to a human cause or mission. Smith's (2007) description of *guerrilla art* is analogous to nursing theorizing. Guerrilla art involves making something that is innovative, flexible, and impermanent, and which derives from the practitioner's inspiration and knowledge as well as out of ethical concern and interaction with one's immediate world. For the nurse, this refers to any of a variety of interactions with patients and their environment that can inform a theory. Furthermore, just as guerrilla art undergoes unique changes when exposed to the elements or is dampened by rain, so too can nurses' theories change in creative ways through their grounded practice with patients.

Practitioners' guerrilla theorizing also resembles what Carver (2002) labeled *theories in the wild* to describe knowledge that is produced in context, interpretive, partial, and always under construction. Carver's (2002) phrase fits the complex and sometimes messy context of nursing practice, where building knowledge is done *with* not just *for* patients and their families and includes the indigenous knowledge of those intimately involved in the health care experience. As Peirce (as cited in Hickman, 2007) expressed, science is not a static body of knowledge but the "concrete life of persons who are working to find out the truth" (p. 247).

Finally, three related concepts—bricoleur, improvisation, and abduction—elaborate on what is meant by *guerrilla theorizing.* They also provide a beginning infrastructure for practice-based theory development.

PRACTITIONER–THEORIST AS BRICOLEUR

Bricoleur is a French term referring to a person who constructs or creates objects or ideas (the *bricolage*) with what is at hand (Manser, 2002). Many sources cite anthropologist Lévi-Strauss's 1966 book, *The Savage Mind,* in describing the bricoleur: one who uses imagination as well as existing knowledge to piece together a diversity of raw materials, objects, methods, philosophies, or ideas that are *at hand* (as opposed to being accessed from outside one's immediate environment) in producing a coherent, new structure (conceptual or concrete) to address a problem. The bricoleur is often described in the context of discussions of qualitative or social research strategies (Denzin & Lincoln, 2003; Kincheloe, 2005).

In their classic description of a bricoleur theorist, Weinstein and Weinstein (1991) depict the bricoleur as one who engages in "disciplined conceptual play" and "seeks generality through particularity" (p. 161). Similarly, practice-based theories are constructed from the particular experiences of patients and nurses but are also *symbolic* constructions (Kaplan, 1964) that therefore reach out to a more general meaning beyond the data. Gobbi (2005) applied the term to describe the everyday work of nurses as both intellectual and technical bricoleurs who adeptly cobble together a variety of elements at hand to formulate a theoretical framework for action. Thus, the unconventional, resourceful, action-oriented, synthetic approach of the bricoleur pertains to the nurse as both practitioner and theorist.

IMPROVISATION

Theory development in nursing practice shares a main characteristic, improvisation, with two unlike occupations, wildland firefighter and jazz musician. Improvisation involves creation of something out of preexisting elements, in the moment and in the natural setting. Weick's (2001) study of wildland firefighting and naturalistic decision making (NDM) demonstrated the importance of improvisation in NDM theorizing-in-action. Improvisation requires discipline and depth of experience as well as "unprogrammed" challenges. He also found that it was more effective to put forth loosely developed hunches than firm hypotheses (typically done in theorizing), which constrain creative thinking. Relevant to theorizing, Weick found that this form of thinking was understood more appropriately as a process of *sense making* than as decision making.

In reference to jazz, a story is told about the iconic jazz musician and composer Miles Davis, who was known for hiring very capable musicians. Just prior to a recording session, instead of handing out the standard charts of music, he gave each musician small pieces of paper with a few musical notes on them, and said, "This is your part." His intent was to create spontaneity yet have the musicians reach beyond themselves and the written music. His approach allowed for artistic freedom while adhering to rules of music theory. This combination of art and theory kept the performance fresh for the musicians and audience while generating a cohesive sound.

Similarly, the practitioner scholar may be able to produce cohesive structures of knowledge called *theories* through a combination of rules of science and artful application of patterns of knowing in their work with patients. Just as improvisation involves balance between disciplinary rules and personal creativity, theory development is a science and an art.

ABDUCTIVE REASONING

The two widely known forms of logic, Aristotle's deductive syllogistic logic and Bacon's inductive logic, are insufficient for theory development. Abduction, a creative form of logic initially described by 20th-century philosopher of science Charles Peirce, plays an integral role in the discovery processes of theory development (Magnani, 2001; Yu, 2001). Abduction is a process of formulating plausible explanations from empirical observations and other knowledge sources. Abductive reasoning requires boldness and creativity. It is *ampliative* in that this form of reasoning expands beyond the information at hand. As theories "deal with . . . entities that are invisible" (Yu, 2001, p. 281), they cannot posit ideas directly from the observed phenomena; guessing or taking conceptual leaps is required.

Abductive reasoning is found repeatedly in descriptions of thinking patterns that underlay theory-development strategies: For example, there is Popper's (1962/1965) concept of *conjecture* in putting forth theory testing ideas; Glaser's (1978) *conceptual leaps* deemed necessary in the discovery of grounded theory, and the process of *puz-zling* (Lipshitz, 2001; Walsh, Moss, Lawless, McKelvie, & Duncan, 2008), which favors puzzle seeking over problem solving and employs action theory to develop knowledge in a professional practice.

Typically, abduction is described as useful in situations where knowledge and protocol are lacking and where solutions are neither clear-cut nor easily solved. More specifically, abduction is a strategy for producing new knowledge (theory), whereby the nurse applies creative insight and knowledge to generate and prioritize potential explanations for the problem at hand. With abduction, the experience or observation occurs first, followed by generation of hypotheses or potential explanations. To get beyond merely solving a problem and into theorizing, nurses need to entertain *why* something is or might be occurring or why an intervention works. Nursing science is about explaining as well as describing. Theories deliver in terms of providing scientific descriptions and explanations. Theories, within varying scopes, deliver on this.

Abduction is garnering increasing attention as a way of thinking theoretically in practice environments. In Kathryn Montgomery's (2006) book, *How Doctors Think*, the journalist promoted abductive thinking as the process underlying physicians' clinical judgment and theorizing for individual cases. Similarly, Hands (2001), as an economist, appropriated Peirce's abduction for his own profession, identifying it as an economics methodology. He stated that a good economist thinks abductively and posited that abductive inferences seem to be the "main 'stuff' of good science . . . [representing] the explanatory hunches and the creative insights that are the mainstay of successful scientific practice" and what is "truly novel and knowledge expanding about human inquiry" (p. 224). He also concludes that abduction may apply to other professions.

NETS OF NURSING KNOWLEDGE

Popper's (1934/1968) epigraph to his 1934 book, *The Logic of Scientific Discovery*, is a maxim by the 18th-century philosopher Novalis: "Theories are nets: only he who casts will catch" (p. 11). Popper elaborated later in his book: "Theories are nets cast to catch what we call 'the world': to rationalize, to explain, and to master it. We endeavour to make the mesh ever finer and finer" (p. 59). His statement reflected the significant influence of theories on translating our observations into meaning and action. However, there is another net metaphor that better represents how practitioners interact with theories today.

This net metaphor was inspired by a book about the roles of women in prehistory (Adovasio, Soffer, & Page, 2007). In one chapter, the authors describe life in Late Paleolithic society 26,000 years ago, where net hunting was a communal affair. The women constructed the nets on the run, adjusting the mesh bigger and smaller to accommodate the varying sizes of life forms available, from large mammals to birds and even insects. Unlike Popper's fishing net that is tossed out repeatedly and mechanically to catch and then master every bit of an unchanging reality, practice-based nursing theories are conceived to be more like the women's traveling nets, constructed on the go within a context and a community, and organic—capable of diversity and adaptation to the current situation, and evolving through interactions with the complex, changing environment.

Theories developed in action are more responsive to the changing needs of a situation. Weick's (2001) firefighter research revealed that *thinking in action* or thinking by taking action, in contrast to *thinking and acting,* was what produced effective knowledge. Magnani (2001) expanded his idea of theoretical abduction to emphasize *manipulative* abduction, a *thinking through doing* in contrast to thinking *about* doing (p. 309).

Action is a reality of practice. So, although practitioners may face challenges in practice-based theory development, their action orientation likely provides distinct advantages over traditional approaches to theorizing. "Scientific creativity is sharpened, not dulled, by rubbing against the whetstone of reality" (Raymo, 2006, p. 72).

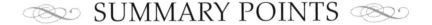

SUMMARY POINTS

1. Acknowledging the practicing nurses as *theorist* marks a new path of knowledge and theory development that can expand our repertoire of strategies for knowledge production in nursing.

2. Theories and theorizing are embedded in practice, as many scholars have attested to the potential for theory development among practitioners.

3. Historical trends in theory development span from Nightingale's empiricism, to Peplau's postpositivism, to Rogers's intermodernism.

4. Methods and tools of clinical inquiry that are potentially useful to practitioners in generating theory include the following: grounded theory methodology, clinical reasoning, structured reflection, participatory action research, and clinical conceptual frameworks.

5. Less conventional methods for theory innovation include guerilla theorizing, improvisation, and abductive reasoning.

6. Although practitioners may face challenges in practice-based theory development, their action orientation may provide distinct advantages over traditional approaches to theorizing.

QUESTIONS FOR REFLECTION

1. In thinking about your work in nursing, what experiences have you had that triggered a new idea you would like to pursue?

2. Of the various strategies in the article for thinking theoretically, which one best fits your style of thinking or working? Does this strategy help you balance "following the rules" with your "personal creativity" in building knowledge?

3. Does the notion of guerrilla theorizing relate to the way you link knowledge to your nursing practice?

4. How might guerrilla theorizing or other strategies be used in a research project?

5. Do you think that practicing nurses are interested in learning ways to develop knowledge and theories in practice? Are there barriers to doing this in practice? What resources would be helpful?

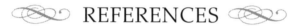 REFERENCES

Adovasio, J. M., Soffer, O., & Page, J. (2007). *The invisible sex: Uncovering the true roles of women in prehistory.* New York, NY: Smithsonian.

Barker, P. (1999). *The philosophy and practice of psychiatric nursing.* Edinburgh, United Kingdom: Churchill Livingstone.

Carper, B. A. (1978). Fundamental patterns of knowing in nursing. *Advances in Nursing Science, 1,* 13–23.

Carver, C. F. (2002). Structures of scientific theories. In P. Machamer & M. Silberstein (Eds.), *The Blackwell guide to the philosophy of science* (pp. 55–79). Malden, MA: Blackwell.

Chaiklin, H. (2004). Problem formulation, conceptualization, and theory development. In A. R. Roberts & K. R. Yeager (Eds.), *Evidence based practice manual: Research and outcome measures in health and human services* (pp. 95–101). New York, NY: Oxford University Press.

Chinn, P. L., & Kramer, M. K. (2015). *Knowledge development in nursing: Theory and process* (9th ed.). St. Louis, MO: Elsevier/Mosby.

Cowling, W. R. (2007). A unitary participatory vision of nursing knowledge. *Advances in Nursing Science, 30,* 61–70.

Denzin, N. K., & Lincoln, Y. S. (2003). *Collecting and interpreting qualitative materials* (2nd ed.). Thousand Oaks, CA: Sage.

Doane, G. H., & Varcoe, C. (2005). Toward compassionate action: Pragmatism and the inseparability of theory/practice. *Advances in Nursing Science, 28*, 81–90.

Ellis, R. (1969). Practitioner as theorist. *American Journal of Nursing, 69*, 1434–1438.

Fawcett, J., Watson, J., Neuman, B., Walker, P. H., & Fitzpatrick, J. J. (2001). On nursing theories and evidence. *Journal of Nursing Scholarship, 33*, 115–119.

Fuller, S. (2000). *Thomas Kuhn: A philosophical history of our times.* Chicago, IL: University of Chicago Press.

Glaser, B. G. (1978). *Theoretical sensitivity.* Mill Valley, CA: Sociology Press.

Gobbi, M. (2005). Nursing practice as bricoleur activity: A concept explored. *Nursing Inquiry, 12*, 117–125.

Hands, D. W. (2001). *Reflection without rules: Economic methodology and contemporary science theory.* Edinburgh, United Kingdom: Cambridge University Press.

Hickman, L. A. (2007). *Pragmatism as post-postmodernism: Lessons from John Dewey.* New York, NY: Fordham University Press.

Kaplan, A. (1964). *The conduct of inquiry: Methodology for behavioral science.* New York, NY: Thomas Y. Crowell.

Kincheloe, J. L. (2005). On to the next level: Continuing the conceptualization of the bricolage. *Qualitative Inquiry, 11*, 323–350.

Kuhn, T. S. (1970). *The structure of scientific revolutions* (2nd ed.). Chicago, IL: University of Chicago Press. (Original work published 1962)

Kuiper, R., O'Donnell, S. M., Pesut, D. J., & Turrise, S. L. (2017). *The essentials of clinical reasoning for nurses.* Indianapolis, IN: Sigma Theta Tau International.

Lévi-Strauss, C. (1966). *The savage mind.* Chicago, IL: University of Chicago Press.

Lipshitz, R. (2001). Puzzle-seeking and model-building on the fire ground. In E. Salas & G. Klein (Eds.), *Linking expertise and naturalistic decision making* (pp. 337–345). Mahwah, NJ: Lawrence Erlbaum.

Magnani, L. (2001). Epistemic mediators and model-based discovery in science. In L. Magnani & N. J. Nersessian (Eds.), *Model-based reasoning: Science, technology, values* (pp. 305–329). New York, NY: Kluwer Academic/Plenum.

Manser, J. H. (2002). *The facts on file dictionary of foreign words and phrases.* New York, NY: Checkmark.

Montgomery, K. (2006). *How doctors think: Clinical judgment and the practice of medicine.* New York, NY: Oxford University Press.

Newman, M. A., Sime, A. M., & Corcoran-Perry, S. A. (1991). The focus of the discipline of nursing. *Advances in Nursing Science, 14*, 1–6.

Nightingale, F. (1969). *Notes on nursing: What it is, and what it is not.* New York, NY: Dover. (Original work published 1859)

Parse, R. R. (1987). *Nursing science: Major paradigms, theories, and critiques.* Philadelphia, PA: W. B. Saunders.

Peplau, H. E. (1988). The art and science of nursing: Similarities, differences, and relations. *Nursing Science Quarterly, 1,* 8–15.

Popper, K. R. (1965). *Conjectures and refutations: The growth of scientific knowledge.* New York, NY: Harper Torchbooks. (Original work published 1962)

Popper, K. R. (1968). *The logic of scientific discovery.* New York, NY: Harper Torchbooks. (Original work published 1934)

Raymo, C. (2006). *Walking zero: Discovering cosmic space and time along the prime meridian.* New York, NY: Walker.

Reed, P. G. (1996). Transforming practice knowledge into nursing knowledge—A revisionist analysis of Peplau. *Journal of Nursing Scholarship, 28,* 29–33.

Reed, P. G. (2006). Neomodernism and evidence based nursing: Implications for the production of nursing knowledge. *Nursing Outlook, 54*(1), 36–38.

Reed, P. G. (2008). Practitioner as theorist: A reprise. *Nursing Science Quarterly, 21,* 315–321.

Reed, P. G. (2011). The spiral path of nursing knowledge. In P. G. Reed & N. B. C. Shearer (Eds.), *Nursing knowledge and theory innovation advancing the science of practice* (pp. 1–35). New York, NY: Springer Publishing.

Reed, P. G., & Lawrence, L. A. (2008). A paradigm for the production of practice-based knowledge. *Journal of Nursing Management, 16,* 422–432.

Rogers, M. E. (1970). *An introduction to the theoretical basis of nursing.* Philadelphia, PA: F. A. Davis.

Rolfe, G., & Gardner, L. (2005). Towards a nursing science of the unique: Evidence, reflexivity and the study of persons. *Journal of Research in Nursing, 10,* 297–310.

Schön, D. A. (1983). *The reflective practitioner: How professionals think in action.* New York, NY: Basic Books.

Smith, K. (2007). *Guerilla art kit: Everything you need to put your message out into the world.* New York, NY: Princeton Architectural Press.

Vosniadou, S. (2001). Mental models in conceptual development. In L. Magnani & N. J. Nersessian (Eds.), *Model-based reasoning: Science, technology, values* (pp. 353–368). New York, NY: Kluwer Academic/Plenum.

Walsh, K., Moss, C., Lawless, J., McKelvie, R., & Duncan, L. (2008). Puzzling practice: A strategy for working with clinical practice issues. *International Journal of Nursing Practice, 14,* 94–100.

Webster's new universal unabridged dictionary. (1996). New York, NY: Barnes and Noble.

Weick, K. E. (2001). Tool retention and fatalities in wildland fire settings: Conceptualizing the naturalistic. In E. Salas & G. Klein (Eds.), *Linking expertise and naturalistic decision making* (pp. 321–336). Mahwah, NJ: Lawrence Erlbaum.

Weinstein, D., & Weinstein, M. A. (1991). Georg Simmel: Sociological bricoleur. *Theory, Culture & Society, 8,* 151–168.

Whall, A. L., & Hicks, F. D. (2002). The unrecognized paradigm shift in nursing: Implications, problems, and possibilities. *Nursing Outlook, 50,* 72–76.

Yu, Q. (2001). Model-based reasoning and similarity in the world. In L. Magnani & N. J. Nersessian (Eds.), *Model-based reasoning: Science, technology, values* (pp. 275–286). New York, NY: Kluwer Academic/Plenum.

10

Clinical Scholarship: History and Future Possibilities

Rene Love

Scholarly inquiry historically has been housed in university settings with the main responsibility for research and other scholarly activities assigned to academicians (Schlotfeldt, 1992). However, clinical scholarship represents a perspective of scholarly inquiry that extends beyond the traditional practices of science. Understanding the historical context of clinical scholarship provides a foundation for discussing new ways to think about theory and knowledge development in nursing. This chapter focuses on clinical scholarship in nursing, including a historical look at movements related to scholarship. Drawing from these historical perspectives and contemporary events, the future of clinical scholarship, particularly in reference to advanced practice nurses, is presented.

Reflecting on the evolution of clinical scholarship in nursing as well as reviewing the contemporary movements of evidence-based practice (EBP) and translational research may offer insights into ways that practicing nurses can be active participants in the development of nursing knowledge in the 21st century. These areas also provide a context for proposing ideas for the future of clinical scholarship and how doctorally prepared nurses in practice will participate in knowledge development.

DEFINING TERMS

It is helpful to begin our exploration of nursing scholarship by defining a few key terms. The term *scholarship* is often used in publications as a noun without a definition. For example, Boyer (1996) spoke of ". . . clinical practice as a form of scholarship" (p. 1). Scholarship, broadly defined today has been enlarged to extend beyond research-based activities to include various forms of inquiry that integrate theory and practice and build knowledge. A scholar is a learned individual who engages in this inquiry within a particular area of knowledge.

Perspectives about the links of practice to scientific knowledge have evolved over time as evident in the terms used to discuss nursing scholarship and practice (see Table 10.1). The definitions of some terms suggest that while nursing practice was considered to be science based, practice often was not regarded as a context for generating practice knowledge.

Nurses with doctorates have been leading scholars throughout the 20th century, encouraged to contribute to nursing knowledge through research and theory building. In contrast, nurses in practice were encouraged to *utilize* the knowledge generated by nursing scholars to guide practice and to identify nursing problems for nursing scholars to study (e.g., Burns & Grove, 2003). The history of clinical nursing scholarship, beginning with Nightingale, belies traditional belief that the role of practicing nurses is knowledge application and not knowledge generation.

NIGHTINGALE: NURSE EXEMPLAR OF SCHOLARSHIP

Florence Nightingale (1820–1910), founder of professional nursing, embodied nursing scholarship. She was a well-educated woman and consummate scholar. Many name her as the first nurse researcher (e.g., Burns & Grove, 2009; Kelly & Joel, 1996). Nightingale drew from her keen empirical observations, sense of moral commitment, and compilation of impressive statistics and other evidence from her practice to lead reform in care of the sick. She reformed health care of the British Army at Scutari to reduce the mortality rate from 42% to 2.2% and initiated a reform in nursing education with the establishment of the Nightingale Training School for nurses. She was adamant about the importance of careful, accurate observations in practice as a basis for effective nursing care. In fact, she dedicated an entire chapter in her *Notes on Nursing* (Nightingale, 1859/1969) to the importance of accurate observations as a knowledge basis for effective patient care. For example, she wrote:

TABLE 10.1 Terms Used in Describing Relationships Between Nursing Theory, Research, and Practice

Term	Definition
Research	"Diligent, systematic inquiry or investigation to validate and refine existing knowledge and generate new knowledge" (Burns & Grove, 2009, p. 719).
Nursing research	". . . a formal, systematic, and rigorous process of inquiry used to generate and test theories about the health-related experiences of human beings within their environments and about the actions and processes that nurses use in practice" (Fawcett & Garity, 2009, p. 5).
Research-based practice	A "systematic, rigorous, and precise way of translating research findings into practice" (Hamric, Spross, & Hanson, 2009, p. 141). (Note that the word *translate* is used here in its generic meaning, rather than the specific meaning in the term *translational research*, referring to the process of moving research findings into practice.)
Scholarship	Acquisition of knowledge gained through education and research in a specific field or branch.
Clinical scholarship	1. "Knowledge derived from the analysis and synthesis of observations of clients and patients . . . a complex activity that has as its purpose the discovery, organization, analysis, synthesis, and transmission of knowledge resulting from client-oriented nursing practice" (Palmer, 1986, p. 318).
	2. ". . . is an approach that enables evidence-based nursing and development of best practices to meet the needs of clients efficiently and effectively . . . requires the identification of desired outcomes; the use of systematic observation and scientifically-based methods to identify and solve clinical problems. . . ." (Sigma Theta Tau Clinical Scholarship Task Force, 1999a, p. 5).
	3. "a professional value and intellectual process, grounded in curiosity about why our clients respond the way they do and why we, as nurses, do the things we do" (Dreher, 1999, p. 29).
	4. Scholarship is "certain habits of mind" (Diers, 1995, p. 25); modifying the term *scholarship* with the word *clinical* highlights the observational or practice dimension of the scholarly activities, without diminishing the required intellectual rigor (Diers, 1995).

(continued)

TABLE 10.1 Terms Used in Describing Relationships Between Nursing Theory, Research, and Practice (*continued*)

Term	Definition
Scholarship of practice (application)	Research skills to test clinical knowledge and new practice strategies (American Association of Colleges of Nursing, 1999).
Evidence-based practice (EBP)	1. "... is the deliberate and critical use of theories about human beings' health-related experiences to guide actions associated with each step of the nursing process" (Fawcett & Garity, 2009, p. 8) broader than research utilization.
	2. "... the integration of individual clinical expertise with the best available external clinical evidence from systematic research" (Sackett, Rosenberg, Gray, Haynes, & Richardson, 1996, p. 71).
	3. EBP stresses use of research findings as well as other sources of credible facts, information, or data (Stetler et al., 1998).
Translational research	1. Research to apply scientific discoveries in practical applications, in order to improve human health (Grady, 2010).
	2. "A study of how research knowledge that is directly or indirectly relevant to health behavior eventually serves the public" (Sussman, Valente, Rohrbach, Skara, & Pentz, 2006, p. 9). May be guided by theories such as diffusion of innovation (Rogers, 2003).

it may safely be said, not that the habit of ready and correct observation will by itself make us useful nurses, but that without it we shall be useless with all our devotion. (Nightingale, 1859/1969, p. 63)

Her emphasis on meticulous observations parallels the emphasis on precise measurement and systematic data collection in contemporary science and nursing research. She reminded readers that the goal of observation (data collection) was to improve care:

In dwelling upon the vital importance of *sound* observation, it must never be lost sight of what observation is for. It is not for the sake of piling up miscellaneous information or curious facts, but for the sake of saving life and increasing health and comfort. (Nightingale, 1859/1969, p. 70)

Despite this emphasis on empirical observation, however, Nightingale also employed critical and theoretical thinking. By this, she formulated empirical generalizations about the data she gathered. The chapter titles in her *Notes on Nursing* can be viewed as a list of some of her major empirical generalizations that provide knowledge for practice in specific areas of nursing care (Reed & Zurakowski, 1996). In particular, Nightingale (1859/1969) advanced theoretical ideas about the relationship of physical and social environmental factors to human health.

Nightingale's words echo ongoing reminders that the goal of clinical observations and nursing scholarship is to build nursing knowledge for improved nursing practice and optimal patient outcomes (Munro, 1997; Grady, 2010). Nightingale's (1859/1969) theories about effective nursing care were detailed in her writings. For example, she wrote that there are five essential points in securing the health of houses: pure air, pure water, efficient drainage, cleanliness, and light. She proposed an inverse relationship between the health of the house and the health of the inhabitants: "Without these (5 concepts), no house can be healthy. And it will be unhealthy just in proportion as they are deficient" (p. 15). Her theory about the relationship between the condition of the house and the health of its inhabitants provided an organizational framework for directing effective nursing care for the sick. These ideas were the predecessors of what were to become two key concepts in nursing's metaparadigm: *environment* and *health.*

Major events regarding nursing knowledge development continued in the 100 years following publication of *Notes on Nursing,* as listed in Table 10.2. The list of selected events reveals that disciplinary changes in research and theory practices occurred relatively independent of each other. The turn of the 20th century brought an increased focus on nursing practice as a source for generating nursing knowledge as well as for applying theory and other forms of knowledge. The importance of scientific knowledge in providing nursing care is a professional legacy that continues on into contemporary nursing (Fawcett & Garity, 2009).

THE EVOLUTION OF CLINICAL SCHOLARSHIP

The term *clinical scholarship* appeared in nursing literature more than 20 years ago to address the intimate relationship between theory, research, scholarship, and practice. Palmer (1986) emphasized the inductive nature of clinical scholarship and its use in improving patient care (Table 10.1). Schlotfeldt (1992) believed that professional nursing depended on clinical scholarship to "generate promising theories for testing that will advance nursing knowledge and insure nursing's continued essential

TABLE 10.2 Selected Research and Theory Events in Nursing Knowledge Development

Year	Key Event
1869	Nightingale publishes *Notes on Nursing: What It Is and What It Is Not* (Nightingale, 1859/1969)
1922	Sigma Theta Tau was founded; a community of nursing scholars (www.nursingsociety.org)
1955	The American Nurses Foundation was founded to fund nursing research (www.anfonline.org)
1950–1960s	Early nursing theorists from Columbia University Teacher's College (Abdellah, 1969; Henderson, 1966; King, 1964; Peplau, 1952) publish their works
1965	American Nurses' Association identified theory development as a significant goal (Meleis, 2007)
1968	First nurse scientist conference on *the nature of science in nursing* (Meleis, 2007)
1970s	Second-generation nursing theorists publish their works (including Rogers, Roy, King, Orem, Neuman), regarded as classic nursing conceptual models (see, e.g., Fitzpatrick & Whall, 1996)
1975	Nursing Theories Conference Group formed out of concern for the need for materials to help nursing students understand and use nursing theories in practice (Meleis, 2012)
1980s	Marked increases in publications focusing on philosophy and theory development and criteria for the critique of extant nursing conceptual models and theories (Nicoll, 1986)
1983	*Image: The Journal of Nursing Scholarship* inaugurated the theme of clinical scholarship with Associate Editor Donna Diers (www.nursingsociety.org/learn-grow/publications/journal-of-nursing-scholarship).
1986	The National Center for Nursing Research (NCNR) established (www.nih.gov/ninr)
1990s	Mid-range theories are distinguished from grand theories (Fawcett, 1993) and there is a marked increase in development of mid-range nursing theories (e.g., Smith & Liehr, 2003)
1992	The NCNR became the National Institute of Nursing Research (www.ninr.nih.gov)
2000	Noted increase in attention to the role of practice in knowledge development (Parker & Smith, 2010)

(continued)

TABLE 10.2 Selected Research and Theory Events in Nursing Knowledge Development (*continued*)	
Year	Key Event
2004	American Association of Colleges of Nursing (2004) position statement on the practice doctorate in nursing distinguishing between the DNP and PhD (www.aacnnursing.org/)
2006	American Association of Colleges of Nursing (2006) essentials of doctoral education for advanced nursing practice (www.aacnnursing .org)
2016	National Organization of Nurse Practitioner Faculties (2016) White Paper: The doctor of nursing practice nurse practitioner as a clinical scholar (www.nonpf.org)

services to humankind" (p. 8). Diers (1995) described scholarship as "certain habits of mind" (p. 25) and said that modifying the term *scholarship* with the word *clinical* highlighted the observational or practice dimension of the scholarly activities without diminishing the intellectual rigor required.

In 1997, Munro introduced a new format in the nursing journal *Clinical Nurse Specialist,* emphasizing a closer relationship between research and practice as clinical scholarship. Munro (1997) wrote:

> I am very excited about the new format of this Journal because research studies will no longer be in a separate section, but incorporated under the relevant heading. This emphasizes the need to view clinical scholarship as basic to excellence in advanced practice. (p. 108)

The implication was that clinical scholarship is the work of nurse researchers and perhaps advanced practice nurses. However, the most important event in promoting clinical scholarship was the presentation of a white paper on clinical scholarship by Sigma Theta Tau International (STTI) at the 35th Biennial Convention (Sigma Theta Tau Clinical Scholarship Task Force, 1999b). This paper is now published online as a resource paper (Sigma Theta Tau Clinical Scholarship Task Force, 1999a).

WHITE PAPER ON CLINICAL SCHOLARSHIP—SIGMA THETA TAU

The board of directors for STTI convened a task force on clinical scholarship serving from 1995 to 1997. The task force continued from 1997 to 1999 with new members, culminating in presentation of a white paper on clinical scholarship at the 35th Biennial Convention. The paper was grounded in the belief that "practice itself is a scholarly undertaking" (Sigma Theta Tau Clinical Scholarship Task Force, 1999b, p. 4) and called for a closer relationship between practice and research. Clinical scholarship was defined as

> an approach that enables evidence-based nursing and development of best practices to meet the needs of clients efficiently and effectively. It requires the identification of desired outcomes; the use of systematic observation and scientifically-based methods to identify and solve clinical problems. (Sigma Theta Tau Clinical Scholarship Task Force, 1999b, p. 5)

The white paper included exemplars of collaborations between academicians and practitioners to address clinical problems in diverse nursing care settings. Clinical scholarship was conceptualized as a means for achieving EBP, and so research and other evidence were used in deciding how to improve practice. However, this initial definition did not explicitly address the role of theory in scholarly practice. In some exemplars, the theoretical basis for the project was identified; in other cases, there was no clear indication of a theoretical foundation. One exemplar of theory-based clinical scholarship presented in the STTI white paper was Friedrich and Dreher's (1999) application of grief theory in a collaborative project between the University of Iowa Hospitals and Clinics and the College of Nursing to study adaptation to severe mental illness. The goal of the project was to improve outcomes for families caring for a family member with mental illness. Researchers and clinicians employed the theory in developing family-centered interventions and in the implementation and evaluation of a new family care model in practice.

CLINICAL SCHOLARSHIP IN PRACTICE

Following the Sigma Theta Tau White Paper, calls for clinical scholarship echoed in every aspect of nursing practice and education. Bell (2003) asked, "Where are the voices from practice who can describe innovative family interventions?" (p. 127). Bell was adamant in her support for clinical scholarship as synthesis of practice knowledge and potential for contribution to theory building in family nursing. She believed that clinical scholarship required concurrent immersion in practice and analysis of the practice itself. She proposed use of Wright and Leahey's (2000) framework for clinical scholarship with distinctions between perceptual (observations), conceptual (analysis), and executive (taking action) skills. Bell (2003) reported using this framework in teaching clinical scholarship for graduate nursing students.

Bell distinguished between clinical research and clinical scholarship as she called for greater participation in clinical scholarship by practitioners themselves. She described the process of *clinical research* as beginning with the researcher understanding a phenomenon, next describing it, and eventually designing and testing interventions. In contrast, she described *clinical scholarship* as beginning with examination of the current practice, next synthesizing practice knowledge (from diverse sources), and including making changes in a theory based on practice (Bell, 2003). She believed clinical scholarship was more complex than nursing research, as it "requires an immersion in clinical practice while simultaneously finding ways to articulate, describe, and analyze what is occurring within clinical practice" (Bell, 2003, p. 128). From her perspective, nurses in practice were essential for the process of clinical scholarship to occur.

CLINICAL SCHOLARSHIP IN NURSING EDUCATION

Scholarship of Students

Nursing educators began to find innovative ways to incorporate learning activities to promote clinical scholarship among their students. For example, Pullen, Reed, and Oslar (2001) reported that faculty created a capstone scholarly paper rather than a comprehensive nursing care plan in response to the emerging importance of clinical scholarship. They adopted Dreher's (1999) definition of clinical scholarship as "a professional value and intellectual process, grounded in curiosity about why our clients respond the way they do and why we, as nurses, do the things we do" (Pullen et al., 2001, p. 1). The authors posited that scholarly writing was an important foundation for clinical scholarship. Students received detailed instructions and mentoring for conducting a review of literature, synthesizing findings, and clinical reasoning, culminating in a doctor of nursing practice (DNP) project paper addressing holistic care of a patient.

The DNP project paper reflects the student's clinical scholarship and synthesis of DNP competencies (American Association of Colleges of Nursing [AACN], 2006). Likewise, the DNP project paper demonstrate evolving clinical scholars' abilities to apply the knowledge obtained during their programs of studies to identify gaps in practice and implementing change. The DNP project is foundational in demonstrating knowledge of not only evaluating best practices, but the ability to translate this knowledge into clinical settings through leadership and interprofessional collaboration. Addressing gaps in health care as a clinical scholar and DNP-prepared leader will have a significant impact on the health care system by improving both access and quality of care to the population.

Scholarship of Faculty

The AACN published definitions of scholarship for the discipline of nursing in the same year (1999) that STTI published its white paper on clinical scholarship. The AACN (1999) defined *scholarship in nursing* as:

> Those activities that systematically advance the teaching, research and practice of nursing through rigorous inquiry that 1) is significant to the profession, 2) is creative, 3) can be documented, 4) can be replicated or elaborated, and 5) can be peer-reviewed through various methods. (p. 3)

The AACN (1999) document (p. 3) incorporated Boyer's (1990) four areas of scholarship in academic work:

1. *Scholarship of discovery:* where new and unique knowledge is generated
2. *Scholarship of teaching:* where the teacher creatively builds bridges between his or her own understanding and the students' learning
3. *Scholarship of application:* where the emphasis is on the use of new knowledge in solving society's problems
4. *Scholarship of integration:* where new relationships among disciplines are discovered (Boyer, 1990)

Examples of the *scholarship of discovery* included primary empirical research, historical research, theory development and testing, methodological studies, and philosophical inquiry and analysis. The scholarship of discovery was documented through peer-reviewed publications, presentations, grant awards, and mentorship.

Examples of the *scholarship of teaching* included development of innovative teaching and evaluation methods, program development, learning outcome evaluation, and professional role modeling. The scholarship of teaching was documented in peer-reviewed publications as well as published textbooks, presentations, and recognition as a master teacher (AACN, 1999).

The *scholarship of practice* encompassed all aspects of the delivery of nursing care and focused on the advancement of clinical knowledge in the discipline. Components of scholarship of practice included development of clinical knowledge, professional development, application of technical or research skills, and scholarly service such as development of practice standards. Documentation of scholarship of practice included peer-reviewed publications, presentations related to practice, grant awards, and recognition as a master practitioner (AACN, 1999). This category of scholarship corresponded most closely to nurses' conceptualizations of clinical scholarship.

Examples of the *scholarship of integration* included activities such as integrative reviews of literature, analyses of health policy, and development of interdisciplinary education programs. Integration could also refer to interdisciplinary inquiry. Documentation was similar to documentation of other areas of scholarship, especially publication in peer-reviewed journals (AACN, 1999).

Evaluation of clinical scholarship differs in academia. How is clinical scholarship defined in your institution? Is it defined through the mission statement or is it defined through the promotion and tenure process? Is clinical scholarship supported through a time commitment by the institution?

DNPS AND CLINICAL NURSING SCHOLARSHIP

DNP graduates are expected to generate knowledge and evidence through their practice to improve patient/population health outcomes (AACN, 2006, 2015). As clinical scholars, working collaboratively with interprofessional teams, they utilize their practice sites as opportunities to engage in both inductive and deductive reasoning, integrating clinical experience with theoretical concepts and propositions, to transform health care. The level of clinical scholarship evolves from a novice as a DNP student to that of expert later in the advanced practice nurse's career.

When looking at the current model of the BSN-DNP education, it is important to understand how levels of scholarship and proficiency are aligned. Using Benner's level of proficiency in nursing (1982) and Boyer's (1996) area of scholarship, a trajectory of scholarship through education and application is suggested (Table 10.3).

Boyer's (1996) four areas of scholarship in nursing clinical practice as listed previously are: 1) *Scholarship of discovery,* 2) *Scholarship of integration,* 3) *Scholarship of teaching, and* 4) *Scholarship of application.*

Benner (1982) defines the five levels of proficiency in nursing as follows:

1. *Novice:* no experience

2. *Advanced beginner:* demonstrates marginal acceptable performance

3. *Competent:* (2 to 3 years) can prioritize care based on evidence but lacks speed and flexibility of a proficient nurse

4. *Proficient:* perceives situations as a whole rather than parts and can individualize based on the specific circumstances

5. *Expert:* no longer relies explicitly on analytical principle to connect the situation to an appropriate action and also uses tacit knowledge in what appears as an "intuitive" grasp of the situation

The integration of these models provides a progression of scholarship for DNP students and DNP graduates who are advanced practice registered nurses (APRNs). The BSN-DNP student begins as a novice provider and novice scholar upon entering a program of study, progressing to advanced beginner as knowledge and practice skills are acquired. The progression as a student scholar culminates in the development of the DNP project, which demonstrates the student's ability to synthesize the

TABLE 10.3 DNP Progression of Scholarship

	Discovery	Integration	Teaching	Application
Novice	BSN-DNP student			
Advanced Beginner				
Competent	New DNP graduate			
Proficient				
Expert	Practice and context dependent			

BSN, bachelor of science in nursing; DNP, doctor of nursing practice.

practice doctorate essentials and competencies. Upon graduation, the student is expected to have obtained minimal competencies and knowledge to transition to a practicing provider and clinical scholar. The addition of several years of experience postgraduation leads to a level of proficiency and then expert as a DNP-prepared APRN. Doctorally prepared nurse practitioners will not only become change agents for local sites but be a prominent force in national and global health care changes.

While years of experience may lead to expert clinicians, this level of proficiency may be site- or population-specific as a provider. A move to a new practice environment or different practice population may reverse the progression as a scholar to competent or proficient for a period of time.

DNP ROLE IN CLINICAL SCHOLARSHIP

The term evidence-based practice (EBP) has been widely used for over 20 years as a desired outcome of clinical scholarship activities (Sigma Theta Tau Clinical Scholarship Task Force, 1999a). Sackett et al. (1996) described EBP as the process of integrating individual clinical expertise with the best available external clinical evidence from systematic research and patient-based data and values. EBP differs from "research utilization" in that EBP incorporates the use of more and diverse knowledge sources—including data from the current clinical context rather than limiting the clinician to findings from a given study in determining best practices.

The Institute of Medicine's pivotal report, *Crossing the Quality Chasm* (Kohn, Corrigan, & Donaldson, 2001), showcased EBP as essential in closing the chasm. EBP allows standardization of best practices in health care, diminishing wide variations in health care, thereby supporting quality and safety and improving health outcomes in patient and population care. There are numerous models and frameworks to support the appraisal, application, and translation of research and other sources of evidence into clinical settings by DNP students/graduates.

One such model was developed by Rosswurm and Larrabee (1999) who published a model for change to EBP, supporting a paradigm shift from tradition- and intuition-driven practice to EBP. They noted that this paradigm shift was possible because nurses could access research findings far more easily (such as by the Internet) than in past years but that nurses still had difficulty synthesizing evidence and integrating their work into practice.

Another model is the ACE Star Model which supports the translation of knowledge into practice (Stevens, 2004). The ACE Star Model of Knowledge Transformation (Stevens, 2004) uses five stages to move knowledge and research into clinical practice. These five stages are as follows:

1. Discovery/research (primary research)
2. Evidence summary (synthesis of knowledge)
3. Translation into guidelines (EBP guidelines)

4. Practice integration (translating into practice)

5. Process, outcome, and evaluation (impact on health outcomes of a patient population)

The model not only addresses the stages of knowledge transformation and the steps to move between the stages, but also potential barriers as well as solutions to moving knowledge into practice.

The Knowledge-to-Action Framework (Graham et al., 2006) is a complex, iterative process with the possibility of using the different phases out of sequence if needed. The processes include knowledge creation (inquiry, synthesis, and products/tools) and the action cycle (monitor knowledge use, evaluate outcomes, sustain knowledge use, identify problem/select knowledge, adapt knowledge to local context, assess barriers to knowledge, and select, tailor, implement interventions). Key to this framework is input from stakeholders who are, at minimum, providers and patients in the local site. All of these frameworks create the foundation to moving EBP forward.

Translational research moves research from the bench to the bedside with the overall goal of improving patient/population health. The trajectory of the process is laid out in four stages: T1 research that is also known as bench or basic research; T2 research that will test new research and/or interventions in controlled environments to obtain knowledge about the efficacy of the interventions in an optimal setting; T3 research will explore a variety of ways to apply recommendations or guidelines in real-life settings; and T4 research addresses interventions influencing the health of populations to improve overall global health (Kon, 2008). DNP students and graduates may have opportunities to be involved in T3 research as they utilize current research and evidence to address the gaps in health care.

In order to meet the demand of crossing the chasm and moving the research into practice, the nursing profession needed to close the gap themselves. The DNP degree was designed to build upon the master of science in nursing competencies at a higher level with additional emphasis on quality improvement, leadership, organizational systems, and policy. The DNP graduate will be able to address the gap identified in the health care system related to practice initiatives and improvement in health care by using evidence-based frameworks. The clinical scholar will decrease the historical time frames required to move best practices into local practice sites.

THE FUTURE OF PRACTICE AND CLINICAL SCHOLARSHIP

The topic of clinical scholarship for the DNP continues to be an important dialogue. The most recent attempt at defining DNP as clinical scholars is an executive summary from the National Organization of Nurse Practitioner Faculties (NONPF, 2016). The white paper builds upon such exemplars of academic–clinical collaborations as presented in the 1999 STTI white paper on clinical scholarship.

The Doctor of Nursing Practice Nurse Practitioner Clinical Scholar (NONPF, 2016) white paper supports the improvement in population health and health care outcomes through the translation of evidence into practice by the DNP scholar. The DNP clinician must never be satisfied with the status quo but must be constantly appraising new methods of care to improve practice and outcomes based on both evidence and practice expertise. The DNP exemplifies clinical scholarship through lifelong learning with involvement in clinical practice and an everlasting sense of intellectual curiosity (NONPF, 2016).

The movement toward preparing more practicing nurses with academic degrees at the doctoral level, DNP as well as PhD, is a distinct opportunity to advance knowledge development efforts to include theory through clinical nursing scholarship. Advanced practice nurses who maintain an active practice and fully embody the synergy among practice, research, and theory will advance nursing knowledge as clinical scholars.

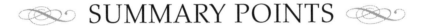# SUMMARY POINTS

1. Nursing has a rich history of clinical scholarship where research, theory, and practice are integrally linked to produce knowledge that promotes quality care and optimal health outcomes.

2. Doctorally prepared nurses in practice are specially educated to not only use but generate and translate knowledge for practice through clinical scholarship.

3. Several frameworks have been developed that are designed to provide guidance in the appraisal, application, and translation of research and other sources of evidence into knowledge for clinical practice.

4. The movement toward preparing more practicing nurses with academic degrees at the doctoral level, DNP as well as PhD, is a distinct opportunity to advance knowledge development efforts through clinical nursing scholarship.

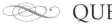# QUESTIONS FOR REFLECTION

1. What activities define your own approach to clinical scholarship?

2. Where are you on the Benner/Boyer table and what would it take to move to the next level?

3. How might contemporary views about clinical scholarship enhance EBP?

4. How can nursing students best learn clinical scholarship and participate in building nursing knowledge?

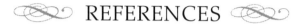 REFERENCES

Abdellah, F. G. (1969). The nature of nursing science. *Nursing Research, 18,* 390–393.

American Association of Colleges of Nursing. (1999, March). *Defining scholarship for the discipline of nursing.* Washington, DC: Author.

American Association of Colleges of Nursing. (2004, October). *AACN position statement on the practice doctorate in nursing.* Washington, DC: Author. Retrieved from http://www.aacnnursing.org/Portals/42/News/Position-Statements/DNP.pdf

American Association of Colleges of Nursing. (2006, October). *The essentials of doctoral education for advanced nursing practice.* Washington, DC: Author. Retrieved from http://www.aacnnursing.org/Portals/42/Publications/DNPEssentials.pdf

American Association of Colleges of Nursing. (2015, August). *The doctor of nursing practice: Current issues and clarifying recommendations: Report from the task force on the implementation of the DNP.* Retrieved from http://www.aacnnursing.org/Portals/42/DNP/DNP-Implementation.pdf?ver=2017-08-01-105830-517

Bell, J. M. (2003). Clinical scholarship in family nursing (editorial). *Journal of Family Nursing, 9*(2), 127–129.

Benner, P. (1982). From novice to expert. *The American Journal of Nursing, 82*(3), 402–407.

Boyer, E. L. (1990). *Scholarship reconsidered: Priorities of the professoriate.* Princeton, NJ: Carnegie Foundation for the Advancement of Teaching.

Boyer, E. L. (1996). Clinical practice as scholarship. *Holistic Nursing Practice, 10*(3), 1–6.

Burns, N., & Grove, S. K. (2003). *Understanding nursing research* (4th ed.). St. Louis, MO: Saunders/Elsevier.

Burns, N., & Grove, S. K. (2009). *The practice of nursing research* (6th ed.). St. Louis, MO: Saunders/Elsevier.

Diers, D. (1995). Clinical scholarship. *Journal of Professional Nursing, 11,* 24–30.

Dreher, M. C. (1999). Clinical scholarship: Nursing practice as an intellectual endeavor. In Sigma Theta Tau Clinical Scholarship Task Force (Ed.), *Clinical scholarship resource paper* (pp. 26–33). Retrieved from https://www.nursingsociety.org/docs/default-source/position-papers/clinical_scholarship_paper.pdf?sfvrsn=4

Fawcett, J. (1993). *Analysis and evaluation of nursing theories.* Philadelphia, PA: F. A. Davis.

Fawcett, J., & Garity, J. (2009). *Evaluating research for evidence-based nursing practice*. Philadelphia, PA: F. A. Davis.

Fitzpatrick, J., & Whall, A. (Eds.). (1996). *Conceptual models of nursing: Analysis and application* (3rd ed.). Stanford, CT: Appleton & Lange.

Friedrich, R. M., & Dreher, M. (1999). Clinical scholarship exemplar: The University of Iowa. In Sigma Theta Tau Clinical Scholarship Task Force (Ed.), *Clinical scholarship resource paper* (pp. 5–6). Retrieved from http://www.nursingsociety.org/docs/default-source/position-papers/clinical_scholarship_paper.pdf?sfvrsn=4

Graham, I. D., Logan, J., Harrison, M. B., Straus, S. E., Tetroe, J., Caswell, W., & Robinson, N. (2006). Lost in knowledge translation: Time for a map? *Journal of Continuing Education in the Health Professions, 26*(1), 13–24.

Hamric, A. B., Spross, J. A., & Hanson, C. M. (2009). *Advanced practice nursing: An integrative approach*. St. Louis, MO: Saunders/Elsevier.

Henderson, V. (1966). *The nature of nursing: A definition and its implications for practice, research, and education*. New York, NY: Macmillan.

Institute of Medicine Committee on Quality of Health Care in America. (2001). *Crossing the quality chasm: A new health system for the 21st Century*. Washington, DC: National Academies Press.

Kelly, L. Y., & Joel, L. A. (1996). *The nursing experience: Trends, challenges, and transitions* (3rd ed.). New York, NY: McGraw-Hill.

King, I. M. (1964). Nursing theory: Problems and prospects. *Nursing Science, 2*, 394–403.

Kon, A. A. (2008). The Clinical and Translational Science Award (CTSA) Consortium and the translational research model. *The American Journal of Bioethics, 8*(3), 58–60.

Meleis, A. I. (2007). *Theoretical nursing: Development and progress* (4th ed.). Philadelphia, PA: Lippincott Williams & Wilkins.

Munro, B. H. (1997). Improving nursing practice through clinical nursing scholarship. *Clinical Nurse Specialist, 11*(3), 108.

Grady, P. A. (2010). Translational research and nursing science. *Nursing Outlook, 58*, 164–166.

National Organization of Nurse Practitioner Faculties. (2016). The doctor of nursing practice nurse practitioner clinical scholar: Executive summary. Retrieved from http://c.ymcdn.com/sites/www.nonpf.org/resource/resmgr/docs/ClinicalScholar FINAL2016.pdf?hhSearchTerms=%22dnp+and+clinical+and+scholar%22

Nicoll, L. H. (Ed.). (1986). *Perspectives on nursing theory*. Boston, MA: Little, Brown.

Nightingale, F. (1969). *Notes on nursing: What it is and what it is not*. New York, NY: Dover. (Original work published 1859)

Palmer, I. S. (1986). The emergence of clinical scholarship: A professional imperative. *Journal of Professional Nursing, 2*, 318–325.

Parker, M. E., & Smith, M. C. (2010). *Nursing theories & nursing practice* (3rd ed.). Philadelphia, PA: F. A. Davis.

Peplau, H. E. (1952). Interpersonal relations in nursing. *The American Journal of Nursing, 52*(6), 765.

Pullen, R. L., Reed, K. E., & Oslar, K. S. (2001). Promoting clinical scholarship through scholarly writing. *Nurse Educator, 26*(1), 81–83.

Reed, P. G., & Zurakowski, T. L. (1996). Nightingale: Foundations of nursing. In J. J. Fitzpatrick & A. L. Whall (Eds.), *Conceptual models of nursing: Analysis and application* (3rd ed., pp. 55–76). Stamford, CT: Appleton & Lange.

Rogers, E. M. (2003). *Diffusion of innovation.* New York, NY: Free Press.

Rosswurm, M. A., & Larrabee, J. H. (1999). A model for change to evidence-based practice. *Image: Journal of Nursing Scholarship, 31*, 317.

Sackett, D. L., Rosenberg, W. M., Gray, J. A., Haynes, R. B., & Richardson, W. S. (1996). Evidence based medicine: What it is and what it isn't. *British Medical Journal, 312*(7023), 71–72.

Schlotfeldt, R. M. (1992). Why promote clinical nursing scholarship? *Clinical Nursing Research, 1*(1), 5–8.

Sigma Theta Tau Clinical Scholarship Task Force. (1999a). Clinical scholarship resource paper. Retrieved from https://www.nursingsociety.org/docs/default-source/position-papers/clinical_scholarship_paper.pdf?sfvrsn=4

Sigma Theta Tau Clinical Scholarship Task Force. (1999b, November). *Clinical scholarship white paper.* Paper presented at the 35th Biennial Convention of Sigma Theta Tau International, San Diego, CA.

Smith, M. J., & Liehr, P. R. (Eds.). (2003). *Middle range theory for nursing.* New York, NY: Springer Publishing.

Stetler, C., Brunell, M., Biuliano, K., Morsi, D., Prince, L., & Newell-Stokes, G. (1998). Evidence-Based practice and the role of nursing leadership. *Journal of Nursing Administration, 28*(7/8), 45–53.

Stevens, K. R. (2004). *ACE Star Model of EBP: Knowledge transformation.* Academic Center for Evidence-Based Practice. The University of Texas Health Science Center at San Antonio. Retrieved from http://nursing.uthscsa.edu/onrs/starmodel/star-model.asp

Sussman, S., Valente, T. W., Rohrbach, L. A., Skara, S., & Pentz, M. A. (2006). Translation in the health professions. *Evaluation & the Health Professions, 29*(1), 7–32.

Wright, L. M., & Leahey, M. (2000). *Nurses and families: A guide to family assessment and intervention* (3rd ed.). Philadelphia, PA: F. A. Davis.

11

Generating Knowledge in Practice: Philosophical and Methodological Considerations

Pamela G. Reed and Barbara B. Brewer

Doctoral nurses have a special synergy for advancing nursing knowledge. They bring learning and insights from the real world of practice and from the theoretical realm of science. Doctoral education of PhD and doctor of nursing practice (DNP) nurses presents new opportunities to build capacity for nursing science. The focus of this chapter is practice-based evidence (PBE) research as an opportunity, particularly for doctoral level practicing nurses, to generate knowledge.

A widespread and continuing concern is that too often the evidence in evidence-based practice (EBP) comes from research using artificially controlled situations and unrepresentative samples that do not translate to the practice setting. Yet, doctoral level practicing nurses, notably DNP nurses, often have been educated into the idea that knowledge development for them is focused on EBP steps of inquiry. This approach does little to *generate* new evidence for practice. Nurses work in environments where they can generate PBE, which goes beyond that of EBP procedures of inquiry. Nursing—buttressed by new thinking in philosophy of science and technology—may outgrow some traditional views about scientific knowledge and constraining beliefs about who can be knowledge producers.

Our goal in this chapter is to guide and encourage nurses to be knowledge generators by engaging in practice-based research (PBR) in settings where they may practice or teach, from point-of-care with patients to system level health care. We present a brief description of PBE research. This is followed by philosophical rationale, which addresses ethical and epistemic considerations for PBR among practicing nurses, including how PBE contrasts with EBP. *Theory* is discussed as the linchpin between conceptual and methodological work in knowledge development. We then present an overview of PBE research methods and close with a model case for generating knowledge in and for practice, and final reflections on building capacity for nursing science.

BRIEF BACKGROUND AND HISTORY OF PBE RESEARCH

PBE research, also referred to as PBR and previously clinical practice improvement, is a research method advocated by Susan Horn (1999) and many other researchers across clinical areas and health care disciplines (Bergstrom, 2008; Brewer, Brewer, & Schultz, 2009; Effgen, McCoy, Chiarello, Jeffries, & Bush, 2016; Gerdle, Molander, Stenberg, Stålnacke, & Enthoven, 2016; Girard, 2008; Green, 2006, 2008; Larson, 2008; Leeman & Sandelowski, 2012; McDonald & Viehbeck, 2007; Salmon & Young, 2013; Westfall, Mold, & Fagnan, 2007; Zimmerman, Domb, Brewer, & Johnson, 2011). PBE research is designed to examine effectiveness of interventions, and their costs and risks within the clinical practice setting. This research method is more practical than the gold standard randomized controlled trials (RCTs), because it allows researchers to evaluate the results of their treatments within the natural environment of clinical practice rather than in an artificially restrictive environment in which attempts are made to remove all extraneous variables through strict inclusion and exclusion requirements of study participants.

DISTINCTIONS BETWEEN EFFICACY AND EFFECTIVENESS—EBP AND PBE

The distinction between efficacy research and effectiveness research is relevant to PBR encouraged in this chapter. RCTs require strict controls in order to establish efficacy of treatments. But interventions found to be efficacious are not necessarily effective across diverse populations and situations. Results may not be transferable to the clinical setting where unexpected factors often intervene and practitioners'

approaches may not exactly match the experimental protocol tested for efficacy. In addition, the required controls of the RCT restrict the evaluation to a group of individuals who have little similarity to patients whom practitioners encounter in their daily practice. Last and importantly, the RCT often requires considerable cost, time, and resources not offset by patient and nursing benefits from the studies.

Horn, Gassaway, Pentz, and James (2010) make the point that the types of individuals who are participating in the RCTs where treatment efficacy is determined are not typical of the patients who clinicians face in their daily practice. What might be effective in participants who participate in rigorously controlled environments may not be so in patients who have comorbid conditions, are of a different age, or are taking other medications to treat other conditions.

Horn and her colleagues have cogently argued for the relevance of PBR designs to overcome the limitations of RCTs while producing knowledge that is relevant to frontline clinicians. It is possible to conduct research that captures more of the complexities of nursing practice and patients' health experiences at the point of care. The evidence and theories indicate that generalizability is not an appropriate goal for research into nursing interventions for the complex health care needs of individuals and populations; more desirable are research approaches that account for relevant factors (patient, caregiver, contextual, care approach, expected outcomes) and their interrelationships rather than control for their effects in artificial ways (Institute of Medicine, 2001; Sidani, Doran, & Mitchell, 2004).

PHILOSOPHICAL PERSPECTIVES

Official documents on doctoral nursing education endorse rigorous knowledge-building research primarily for PhD nurses. Currently, approximately 1% of nurses are developing new knowledge for the remaining 99%. This division in knowledge-generation labor may not be sustainable in light of looming shortages in doctoral nurses and faculty that translate into a shortage of nursing knowledge. In addition to this practical concern of a knowledge shortage, there are ethical and epistemic reasons for educating and empowering practicing nurses for leadership roles in knowledge production. It is time to build upon the achievement of visionary educational leaders, who so ably and aptly established the practice doctorate in nursing, to embrace new thinking about knowledge production in practice. Building capacity for nursing knowledge will require leadership and participation of both PhD and DNP nurses in research, in academic and practice settings.

ETHICAL CONSIDERATIONS

Results from research regarding determinants and correlates of the differentiation between DNP and PhD roles in knowledge development raise concern about inclusion. This academic degree differentiation may foster hierarchies in faculty status and available research resources, feelings among DNP nurses of marginalization and being undervalued and PhD nurse perceptions that DNP nurses are not prepared to develop knowledge-generating research, contribute to nursing scholarship, and be successful in tenure-track positions (Dreher, Glasgow, Cornelius, & Bhattacharya, 2012; Staffileno, Murphy, & Carlson, 2017). In a study of 340 nurses in which PhD and DNP faculty perceptions about DNP faculty roles were compared, Udlis and Mancuso (2015) found that over twice as many DNP as PhD nurses agreed that DNP faculty contributed to nursing scholarship, and four times as many DNP as PhD nurses agreed that DNP faculty were capable of developing knowledge-generating research. Whether DNP nurses experience a form of epistemic injustice related to perceived lack of knowledge in academia is not clear, although this has occurred in practice settings (Reed & Rishel, 2015).

Doctoral level practitioners in other professions (e.g., MD, PharmD) are considered knowledge producers and engage in inquiry beyond EBP steps of problem solving. Building knowledge to keep up with needs for new knowledge about health, emerging health problems, and changes in health care delivery requires use of research methods that generate new evidence. Potempa, Redman, and Anderson (2008) found, unsurprisingly, that faculty colleagues in medicine and public health outpaced nursing in federal funding. Some of their conclusions pointed to the role of the DNP nurse in expanding nursing capacity for clinical scholarship. DNP nurses are rapidly assuming faculty roles. They must be able to lead knowledge production efforts and compete for research funding with confidence and respect as do other practice doctorate faculty in health sciences centers and academia.

EPISTEMIC CONSIDERATIONS

Epistemic considerations refer to issues concerning the relevance and validity of knowledge, and how nurses generate and warrant disciplinary knowledge in practice. A broadening in focus beyond EBP to PBE can enhance the epistemic qualities of knowledge used in practice. EBP procedures as a form of inquiry are important but insufficient for providing knowledge for practice. The *epistemic limitations of EBP* are familiar, and include the following:

- Weak link to theory and theory-informed perceptions about practice problems and health care approaches (Karnick, 2016)

- Inadequate integration of point-of-care clinical expertise and patient preferences (Taylor, Priefer, & Alt-White, 2016)

- Neglect of addressing how "research evidence interacts with clinical experience, the nurse's situational knowledge and clinical expertise, patient and family experiences and preference, and contextual factors" (Rycroft-Malone et al., 2004, p. 86)

- Failure to account for knowledge from sources in nursing ways of knowing (Avis & Freshwater, 2006)

- Inability to promote scientific rigor in clinical decision making and false claim of ruling out influence of intuition in knowledge (Devisch & Murray, 2009)

- Promotes misleading confidence that there is one problem and one best treatment

Several of the limitations of EBP for patient-centered care are summed in a critique by philosopher of science Borgerson (2009) who argued that EBP is unjustified in its approach to knowledge in that it restricts practice with patients and "diverts attention from many legitimate sources of evidence."

The EBP movement (Sackett, Rosenberg, Gray, Haynes, & Richardson, 1996) arose in medicine in response to concerns about the lack of scientific rigor in medical practice. Similarly, PBR arose to address limitations of evidence obtained through certain forms of scientific inquiry such as RCTs and systematic reviews based on these studies that often control for or overlook practice-related factors regarded as having epistemic value. In contrast, PBE research systematically incorporates into its methods practice-relevant factors, for example, health care provider, patient, and family knowledge and perspectives, and social, situational, and other contextual variables. These are considered to have epistemic value in that they have a significant role in explaining or influencing the problem or process under study, and in building knowledge that is valid. PBR has an underlying epistemology that expands upon the hierarchy of evidence of the EBP model as to what methods warrant scientific knowledge. The research on which EBP is based is usually conducted by scientists who are removed from the practice setting and who focus on epistemic values of objectivity and generalization. Treatment efficacy (*does the treatment cause an effect?*) rather than treatment effectiveness (*does the treatment work effectively and efficiently in the practice context of other intervening factors?*) is the focus of RCTs.

Understanding these limitations will help nursing make the most appropriate use of EBP methods. While EBP procedures can be useful in identifying and organizing research results to identify potential approaches to address a clinical problem, EBP is not a translational strategy in itself; translation research is still needed to determine the effectiveness of and to refine translation strategies. Further, because this research is based on evidence drawn from EBP research, it is likely to be less effective for practice than results generated from PBR.

In conclusion, EBP procedures alone cannot warrant nursing knowledge for practice. Nursing epistemology, like that of other scientific disciplines, requires rigorous research (quantitative and qualitative), along with knowledge obtained through other patterns of knowing, to warrant knowledge upon which nurses base their health care of human beings, families, and communities. PBE research results can increase understanding of complex and unique experiences and needs of patients—in keeping with nursing's philosophy of practice.

A PHILOSOPHICAL PERSPECTIVE FOR PRACTICE-BASED KNOWLEDGE PRODUCTION

A new philosophy of science perspective has emerged over the past two decades that is particularly aligned with and supports the PBE research for generating knowledge. The scientific goal is not based on the positivist interest in obtaining the one truth of the matter, but rather the pragmatist interest in obtaining knowledge to solve problems and promote human well-being (e.g., Dewey, 1938; Longino, 2002). This philosophical perspective claims that contextual values (social, practical, ethical) as well as cognitive (rational, logical) have epistemic value in knowledge development and application. This is a shift from traditional ideals of science for value-free, decontextualized, objective inquiry. As such, for example, patient values and preferences and nursing insights are not extrinsic to what is deemed as scientific evidence; they constitute variables that directly influence what researchers (and practitioners) regard as the "truth" or evidence, at least for the practice situation and problem under study. The methods of PBE research and the subsequent translation and application of its use of this evidence in nursing practice account for this array of values and variables that can make a difference in nursing care. And these factors have a role in both science and practice—from the researcher's methods and design of a study to the practitioner's interactions and decision approaches with patients and families.

The nature of nurses' work requires knowledge produced out of research relevant to the intricacies of the situation at hand. Nurses work in contexts that are both determinate and indeterminate. *Determinate* situations are more or less routine and hold established shared understandings about health care for expected and unexpected problems. *Indeterminate* situations have elements that are emergent and not so clearly defined in the context, and with stakeholders who may have differing values about what is relevant in assessing and addressing a problem. Indeterminate situations evoke inquiry (Dewey, 1938). PBR is useful in gaining knowledge of what is happening (descriptive methods) and why (explanatory methods), so that informed decisions can be made and approaches or interventions can be designed in a way that is timely while accounting for both the routine and unpredictable factors of practice.

Within this practice-based philosophical perspective, the producer of scientific knowledge is not the individual but a community of knowers in which decisions are negotiated, not dictated. This notion of a community of inquiry is also reflected in the work of Gibbons et al. (1994) who distinguished between two modes of knowledge production. Mode 1 knowledge production employs traditional forms of scientific inquiry, distinguishing between the scientist and the practitioner and valuing objectivity in knowledge development. Mode 2 knowledge is coproduced by the researcher in participation with a community, and crosses boundaries of disciplinary knowledge. This transdisciplinary nature of Mode 2 knowledge production fits the interprofessional nature of health care practice. Mode 2 knowledge production facilitates effective translation of research knowledge into interdisciplinary practice; it promotes if not requires interactions among many stakeholders—including the knowledge generators, translators, and end users.

However, this philosophy of knowledge production must also champion the unique knowledge and voice of nurses, as having irreplaceable and essential insights into patient care and health care delivery. A particular strength of practice-based approach to knowledge development is that it engages the voices of all stakeholders in knowledge development (e.g., Glass & Newman, 2015).

Doctorally prepared practicing nurses are often in a prime position for leading practice-relevant research. At one level, nurses as evidence-based practitioners are appraisers of existing results from research, which they apply in their practice, consistent with earlier recommendations from the American Association of Colleges of Nursing (AACN, 2006b). Moreover, recent recommendations (AACN, 2015) also acknowledge the importance of research-based knowledge-generating roles of DNP nurses. Doctorally prepared practicing nurses are members of transdisciplinary patient care teams and often stand at the intersection of where planning, implementation, and evaluation of care can occur. Here is where PBE research, done in real time, is especially advantageous within a health care context that is emergent, dynamic, and complex. PBE research is designed to address emergent as well as ongoing problems by connecting with a community for identifying problems and interpreting findings. Further, a practice-based view of knowledge inspires innovative research methods (Kuhn & Jackson, 2008).

In summary, this philosophical view integrates contextual and ethical values into an intermodernist (see Chapter 2, this book) approach to science, knowledge, and evidence. That is, knowledge is regarded as a product of social as well as individual epistemological processes, whereby scientific inquiry occurs in a pluralistic context of multiple values, influences, and ways of knowing from empirical to sociopolitical. It supports PBR methods that are not only responsive to the immediate need of evidence to solve current problems, but that also uphold scientific rigor to generate reliable and valid evidence for theory-based knowledge.

FACILITATING KNOWLEDGE PRODUCTION IN RESEARCH: THEORY INNOVATION

An important dimension of knowledge development is its connection to theoretical thinking. All the research methods and data in the world cannot generate knowledge without the conceptual innovation called "theory." Theory is a tool or strategy, not unlike the tools and strategies of research methods.

As indispensable tools of knowledge production, theories facilitate the entire knowledge development process for practice—from determining what is the proper problem to study and the initial conceptualization of the problem, to identifying relevant variables and how to measure them, to interpreting the meaning and application of the results, and then translating the findings and designing the interventions, interactions, practice guides, and other approaches. Theory also guides the evaluation and refining of these practice approaches. Theories most importantly provide descriptions of phenomena and explanations for what is going on.

Theory represents various types of conceptual structures of different levels of scope and specificity, ranging from conceptual models and frameworks to situation-specific or microtheories. Each can be useful depending on the stage, purpose, and type of research. For example, exploratory research uses a more general theory, called a conceptual framework, whereas descriptive research and explanatory research employ middle range theory that specifies the variables and their relationships

Broadly, then, theory provides a lens from the beginning to end of the inquiry, guiding the nurse in seeing what the significant issues are so as to not be distracted by lesser problems. Because of the complexity of variables that are potentially relevant in PBR, theory is especially important in initially providing a lens to frame the significant variables of a problem for inquiry. A theory will become more specified with research results, integrating findings and revealing what is known and what are the gaps or inconsistencies in knowledge.

Developing theory is both a creative and a systematic process; various strategies are used, more or less, to guide the theory development process. Theories are also based on assumptions that reflect social and personal values, worldviews, beliefs, and sociopolitical factors—all of which can influence the research process and exist within PBR contexts. As structures of human creativity, knowledge, and values, theories are subject to analysis and critique for scientific and pragmatic adequacy. Importantly, they are adaptable and open to change.

Theories gain empirical adequacy by integrating results obtained across studies over time in a meaningful way. Theories should be consistent with existing research results, yet be open to critique and change, modification, or transformation based on new findings and other changes in the practice context—all qualities of a theory that are particularly relevant in PBR. Knowledge in the form of theory can enhance *understanding* or *prediction*, even in the absence of *explanation*, where explanation involves knowledge of underlying processes or mechanisms of why events are connected or cause certain outcomes. The complexity of the world makes it difficult for any theory to both fully explain and predict events. Theories also expose gaps and inconsistencies in knowledge.

To conclude, the knowledge embedded in a theory is not narrow like that found in problem-solving solutions. Rather, because theory is both supported by empirical work and of a higher level of abstraction, it can reach across time and place to provide knowledge for other similar situations. Dewey (1938) expressed this abstract yet pragmatic nature of theories in explaining that events hold a "double life"; there is the concrete life we experience and an abstract level of meaning. A critical part of inquiry is theorizing, to link the concrete observed in practice and discovered in research, to significance and meaning. Practice knowledge is the outcome of inquiry, connecting theory and experience, and transforming indeterminate situations into determinate situations. Theory, in the hands of the expert nurse, facilitates transfer of abstract knowledge for practical guidance.

PBE RESEARCH METHODS

Doctorally prepared practicing nurses are in prime positions to lead practice-oriented research to generate knowledge that addresses various clinical concerns and problems. In virtue of the nature of their work, nurses have intimate connections to patients, their families and community, and the health care system. These connections—a kind of indigenous knowledge—coupled with research and theory, can inform and facilitate nursing practices to enhance patient outcomes.

Knowledge generated from this research then contributes to the evidence nurses use to promote health and improve patient outcomes across a variety of health care settings, from the bedside to hospital unit, and from in-home care to the clinic and community. Nursing knowledge is also needed to minimize untoward consequences of patient care delivered within complex environments to individuals with ever more complicated and uncertain interactions among comorbid conditions.

This research may range from identifying and describing potentially significant factors in nursing care, or examining relationships between specific variables proposed to play a role in patient well-being, to evaluating outcomes resulting from evidence put into practice. Nurses are also in a position to measure outcomes for a population of patients for which they are responsible, which will become more important as we move forward with financial changes and new accountabilities related to accountable care.

EXAMPLES OF DESIGNS
AND METHODS

In PBR, the practice setting is the laboratory for a variety of types of research (observational studies; surveys of providers, patients, and families; analysis of secondary data and electronic health record [EHR] data; and qualitative research) across phases of the research process (exploratory, descriptive, explanatory, and translational or prescriptive). The designs include cohort studies (prospective population-based), case studies, case control (matched sample design), comparative effectiveness, and sometimes RCTs. These designs involve measurement of patient characteristics, process measures, and outcomes (Horn, 1999; Horn & Gassaway, 2007, 2010; Horn et al., 2010). In PBR designs, it is critically important that all variables be specified correctly in order to capture all data relevant to comparing effectiveness across treatments in patients with different characteristics in order to control for initial differences in patients and avoid confounding causes for outcomes of care. Examples of studies using PBE research methods *to evaluate comparative effectiveness* are the following: in postacute care (Horn & Gassaway, 2007), in smoking cessation best practices (Campbell, Ossip-Klein, Bailey, Saul, & North American Quitline Consortium, 2007), in group physical therapy outcomes of acute spinal cord injury patients in inpatient rehabilitation (Zanca et al., 2011), and in pediatric oncology to reduce central line–associated bloodstream infections (Linder, Gerdy, Abouzelof, & Wilson, 2016).

Next, we elaborate on a few designs and methods that are used in PBE research. Most use quantitative data, but qualitative methods can be effectively used too.

Cohort studies have a prospective research design where researchers evaluate if a population of interest develops a disease or an outcome based on hypothesized risks (Polit & Beck, 2017). An example on a larger scale, however, is the Framingham Heart Study, which has been following residents from a city in Massachusetts for decades trying to better understand risk factors associated with developing coronary heart disease or acute myocardial infarctions. Many of the risk factors that we know today are associated with coronary heart disease were learned through this body of research (Long & Fox, 2016). A second well-known and long-running cohort study is the Nurses' Health Study, which is in its third generation and brought to light many risk factors for chronic illness in women such as relationships between estrogen and glaucoma (Dewundara, Wiggs, Sullivan, & Pasquale, 2016), and relationships among body shapes and mortality (Song et al., 2016).

Case-controlled studies are retrospective studies where researchers link phenomena in the present to those which occurred in the past. When designing a case-control study, the researcher tries to match individuals who have a disease or condition with those (control) who do not (Polit & Beck, 2017). Matching is done using demographic data, such as age, gender, and smoking history, with the goal of reducing confounding by including individuals who do not have the disease or condition but are as close as possible to those who have the disease or condition. Examples of case-controlled studies are a study that assessed risk factors for delirium following cardiovascular surgery (CheheiliSobbi et al., 2016) and a second study that examined the association between migraine headaches and restless legs syndrome (Lin et al., 2016).

Nurses are also in an excellent position to work with other clinicians to *design prospective data collection instruments to be able to document care processes* in a standard way (Horn et al., 2010). For example, if a group of primary care providers wished to examine their outcomes related to glucose management in their patients with type 2 diabetes, they may use hemoglobin A1C (Hgb A1C) as an outcome measure that is readily available in the electronic medical record. If evaluating Hgb A1C without understanding differences in the patient's medications, comorbid conditions, physical activity, diet, and other relevant factors associated with glucose control, then spurious conclusions might be made about reasons for control. The DNP, as an expert nurse, can lead the clinical team to ensure all relevant management process indicators, whether they be treatment based such as medications or personally based such as exercise levels and diet, are included in the data collection instrument ensuring that all relevant variables are included in the statistical model that controls for individual patient differences when evaluating outcome (Hgb A1C) levels.

The proliferation of EHRs and digitally available patient data have enabled evaluations of the effectiveness of interventions and other care approaches to be done efficiently and at a much lower cost than what was possible when patient data were unavailable in digital format. EHR data allow large-scale descriptive research studies to be performed, such as cohort (Hammond et al., 2015; Siebens et al., 2016) and case-controlled (Cochran et al., 2013), as well as using the newer data mining approaches that have burgeoned with the emergence of data science (Westra et al., 2016). Research performed using PBE methods uses statistical techniques to control for patient and care differences found in practice using clinical data enabling evaluation in thousands of patients at relatively low cost (Horn et al., 2010).

Qualitative methods can be especially useful in PBR. Nurses use a variety of qualitative methods for achieving different purposes in building or extending evidence. Qualitative methods are used for a variety of research purposes such as the following: identify and describe focal and contextual variables and their relationships to each other; identify and describe diverse characteristics of a patient, group, family, or community; understand the meaning and experience of a situation from individual perspectives; identify desired outcomes and specify parameters of a potential intervention or program; describe psychosocial or structural processes associated with a given health problem; and elucidate potential underlying mechanisms of treatment outcomes. Methods include grounded theory, qualitative descriptive, phenomenology (various types), and ethnography. (For an example of qualitative methods in PBE research, see Leeman & Sandelowski, 2012; Nicholson, Hinden, Biebel, Henry, & Katz-Leavy, 2007.)

A CASE MODEL OF A PBE STUDY

The following is a case example of a practice-based approach to research. It includes the components of identification and rationale of the practice problem, theoretical framework to support the research, the method used to examine the problem, and the outcome of the research.

PRACTICE PROBLEM

A case example of PBR involves evaluating the effectiveness of different oral care processes in preventing ventilator-associated pneumonia (VAP) in critical care patients. Acute care DNPs were noticing that there was variability in the numbers of VAP cases they saw in their practices from month to month. In order to better understand why and to try to mitigate the risk of developing VAP in future patients, they decided to perform a PBE study to evaluate relationships between different oral care treatments and development of VAP.

THEORY

Before beginning their study, they determined that they would use a physiological theory to guide the selection of variables for the study and to put their results into perspective. Based on their theory, they evaluated variables and processes that were associated with removing dental plaque, which has been associated with development of VAP. In order to ensure they captured all care processes before beginning data collection, they asked a group of critical care nurses to list all forms of oral care performed in their unit. The result was application of chlorhexidine gluconate by swabbing the patient's oral cavity twice daily, tooth brushing every 8 hours, and a combination of the two.

From their nursing perspective of the whole person, the nurses also employed a second theory to address the health being more holistically. They used Kolcaba's (2003) comfort theory, which had been tested and refined to include hospital-based outcomes. Use of this theory alerted them to the importance of controlling for selected environmental, sociocultural, psychospiritual, and physical factors that could cause discomfort and stress during the procedure and exacerbate a problem. Controlling for variations in comfort across all participants reduced the varying influences undue discomfort might have on the outcome.

METHOD

In order to determine differences in effectiveness of the three forms of oral care being performed in the critical care unit, the researchers developed a data collection tool that would be used to extract data from the electronic medical record during a specified time period. The data collection tool contained variables related to patient characteristics, such as gender, age, length of stay, diagnosis, reason for ventilator, comorbid conditions, condition of teeth and/or dentures, and lab values. It also contained variables for collection of process variables related to oral care, such as frequency, time of delivery, type (chlorhexidine, tooth brushing, or both) and dose (amount of chlorhexidine, length of tooth brushing) of oral care, and other forms of oral care, such as suctioning. In addition, an observational tool was developed and used during the same time period to record the comfort rating in each of the four theorized areas of comfort care. Analysis indicated no significant differences on each component across participants.

They determined that pneumonia that was identified radiographically and that occurred 48 hours or more following intubation would define the presence of VAP. The sample consisted of all ventilated patients from the previous 2 years who had been intubated during that hospital stay. Analysis involved multivariate logistic regression to control for confounding variables associated with patient characteristics and predict the risk of developing VAP related to the different oral care treatments.

OUTCOME

Upon completion of their analysis, they determined that patients who had teeth brushed consistently had lower odds of developing VAP than those who had chlorhexidine swabs and similar odds to those who had tooth brushing and chlorhexidine swabs. As a result, future oral care treatments eliminated chlorhexidine swabs as an option, which not only simplified care for the nursing staff, but reduced costs by eliminating the need to purchase the oral care kits containing the chlorhexidine swabs.

CONCLUSIONS: BUILDING CAPACITY FOR NURSING KNOWLEDGE

Doctoral nurses in practice are often situated in key positions to lead PBE research. As perhaps the only doctoral level nurses within their organization, whether a community-based practice or an acute care hospital, nurses will be expected to lead efforts to evaluate the effectiveness of care practices by quality improvement or small research projects. Research activities such as these build knowledge, whether at the local level (in a single primary care practice) or at a grander level (across a health care system).

Nurses are the experts of patient-centered care. Doctoral education supports development of this expertise, with preparation in clinical care, theory, leadership, policy, and evidence generation and evaluation among other areas. Educational preparation must continue to enable and empower nurses to broaden their clinical scholarship beyond EBP procedures to engage in PBE research. This includes leading and participating in "measurement of their own patient and process outcomes and measurements within the organization and communities where they practice" (Issel, 2016, p. 73). Doctoral educators of both PhD and DNP nurses are developing curricula that incorporate a variety of increasingly sophisticated methods and designs for PBR with individuals, groups, communities, and systems (e.g., Bloch, Courtney, & Clark, 2016; Magyary, Whitney, & Brown, 2006).

Practicing nurses should not be excluded—by institutional and social factors, or by a lack of education or self-confidence in their role—from fully participating in scientific methods of knowledge production. An integrative review of research indicated that clinical nurses are involved in research from acting as principal investigators, reviewers, mentors, and institutional review board members (Scala, Price, & Day, 2016). In addition, engaging in research is a best practice and enhances uptake of research evidence in practice (Hagan & Walden, 2015).

Some have suggested that the generation of new knowledge in nursing is best done by those who have achieved research-focused doctoral degrees, while those who achieve practice-intensive doctoral degrees translate new knowledge into practice (AACN, 2006a; Buchholz et al., 2013). While this may be true in some situations, rigid adherence to this type of thinking is narrow and prohibits opportunities for nurses to contribute to knowledge development and to build capacity for the advancement of nursing science. The latest recommendations from the AACN (2015) have clarified the knowledge-generating capabilities of the DNP nurse. Doctorally prepared clinicians, PhD or DNP, are especially and uniquely positioned to generate practice-informed knowledge. Ultimately, PBR facilitates better nursing science, theory, and practice by engaging nurses, patients and families, and other health care professionals in knowledge generation that is both timely and relevant to health care.

SUMMARY POINTS

1. PBE research, also referred to as PBR, is an approach that can be used by nurses to generate knowledge in practice, beyond that offered through EPB procedures.

2. Shifts that are occurring in philosophy of science support the movement toward practice-based knowledge generation for patient-centered care.

3. A broadening in focus beyond EBP to PBE can enhance nursing capacity for building practice knowledge, particularly given the limitations of EBP for patient-centered nursing practice.

4. A particular strength of the practice-based approach to knowledge development is that it engages the voices of many stakeholders in knowledge development.

5. As members of transdisciplinary patient care teams, DNPs and other doctorally prepared nurses are at the intersection of care provision and knowledge generation.

6. Theory is an essential conceptual tool for building knowledge through PBR across all phases of the research through translation.

7. PBE research is a cost-effective method for evaluating the effectiveness of treatments within their natural setting.

8. There is a wide variety of research designs nurses can use to conduct PBE research in their own clinical setting.

9. The proliferation of EHRs provides an important source of data to evaluate the effectiveness of care. Leadership of doctorally prepared nurses is needed to transform the available data into meaningful knowledge regarding the effectiveness of clinical practices.

10. Doctoral education for nursing will enable and empower nurses to engage in creative PBR that builds capacity for nursing knowledge.

QUESTIONS FOR REFLECTION

1. Have you noticed or experienced any positive or negative influences for nursing science and practice from the differentiations between PhD and DNP nurses?

2. From your perspective, what are the advantages or challenges of doing PBE research?

3. What advantages does having practice experience provide for building theory and knowledge in nursing? Should nursing practice experience (in some form) be an expectation for those who claim to be developing nursing knowledge?

4. Among the various research designs and methods, do you prefer any particular research design for your own doctoral research approach?

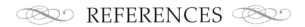 REFERENCES

American Association of Colleges of Nursing. (2006a). *AACN position statement on nursing research*. Retrieved from http://www.aacnnursing.org/Portals/42/News/Position-Statements/DNP.pdf

American Association of Colleges of Nursing. (2006b). *The essentials of doctoral education for advanced nursing practice*. Retrieved from http://www.aacnnursing.org/Portals/42/Publications/DNPEssentials.pdf

American Association of Colleges of Nursing. (2015). *The doctor of nursing practice: Current issues and clarifying recommendations*. Washington, DC: Author. Retrieved from http://www.aacnnursing.org/Portals/42/DNP/DNP-Implementation.pdf?ver=2017-08-01-105830-517

Avis, M., & Freshwater, D. (2006). Evidence for practice, epistemology, and critical reflection. *Nursing Philosophy, 7*, 216–224.

Bergstrom, N. (2008). The gap between discovery and practice implementation in evidence-based practice: Is practice-based evidence a solution? *International Journal of Evidence Based Health, 6*, 135–136.

Bloch, J. R., Courtney, M. R., & Clark, M. L. (Eds.). (2016). *Practice-based clinical inquiry in nursing for DNP and PhD research: Looking beyond traditional methods*. New York, NY: Springer Publishing.

Borgerson, K. (2009). Valuing evidence: Bias and the evidence hierarchy of evidence-based medicine. *Perspectives in Biology and Medicine, 52*(2), 218–233.

Brewer, B. B., Brewer, M. A., & Schultz, A. A. (2009). A collaborative approach to building the capacity for research and evidence-based practice in a community hospital. *Nursing Clinics of North America, 44*(1), 11–25.

Buchholz, S. W., Budd, G. M., Courtney, M. R., Neiheisel, M. B., Hammersla, M., & Carlson, E. D. (2013). Preparing practice scholars: Teaching knowledge application in the Doctor of Nursing Practice curriculum. *Journal of the American Association of Nurse Practitioners, 25*(9), 473–480.

Campbell, H. S., Ossip-Klein, D., Bailey, L., Saul, J., & North American Quitline Consortium. (2007). Minimal dataset for quitlines: A best practice. *Tobacco Control, 16*(Suppl. 1), 16–20.

CheheiliSobbi, S., van den Boogaard, M., Slooter, A. J., van Swieten, H. A., Ceelen, L., Pop, G., . . . Pickkers, P. (2016). Absence of association between whole blood viscosity and delirium after cardiac surgery: A case-controlled study. *Journal of Cardiovascular Surgery, 11*(1), 132. doi:10.1186/s13019-016-0517-9

Cochran, A., Thuet, W., Holt, B., Faraklas, I., Smout, R. J., & Horn, S. D. (2013). The impact of oxandrolone on length of stay following major burn injury: A clinical practice evaluation. *Burns, 39*(7), 1374–1379.

Devisch, I., & Murray, S. J. (2009). "We hold these truths to be self-evident": Deconstructing "evidence-based" medical practice. *Journal of Evaluation in Clinical Practice*, *16*, 950–954.

Dewey, J. (1938). The pattern of inquiry. In J. Dewey (Ed.), *Logic, the theory of inquiry*. New York, NY: H. Holt.

Dewundara, S. S., Wiggs, J. L., Sullivan, D. A., & Pasquale, L. R. (2016). Is estrogen a therapeutic target for glaucoma? *Seminars in Ophthalmology, 31*(1–2), 140–146.

Dreher, H. M., Glasgow, M. E., Cornelius, F. H., & Bhattacharya, A. (2012). A report on a national study of doctoral nursing faculty. *Nursing Clinics of North American, 47*, 435–453.

Effgen, S. K., McCoy, S. W., Chiarello, L. A., Jeffries, L. M., & Bush, H. (2016). Physical therapy-related child outcomes in school: An example of practice-based evidence methodology. *Pediatric Physical Therapy, 28*(1), 47–56.

Gerdle, B., Molander, P., Stenberg, G., Stålnacke, B., & Enthoven, P. (2016). Weak outcome predictors of mulitmodal rehabilitation at one-year follow-up in patients with chronic pain—a practice based evidence study from two SQRP centers. *BioMed Central Musculoskeletal Disorders, 17*. doi:10.1186/s12891-016-1346-7

Gibbons, J., Limoges, C., Nowotny, H., Schwartzman, S., Scot, P., & Trow, M. (1994). *The new production of knowledge: The dynamics of science and research in contemporary societies*. Thousand Oaks, CA: Sage.

Girard, N. J. (2008). Practice-based evidence. *Association of periOperative Registered Nurses Journal, 87*(1), 15–16.

Glass, R., & Newman, A. (2015). Ethical and epistemic dilemmas in knowledge production: Addressing their intersection in collaborative, community-based research. *Theory and Research in Education, 13*(1), 23–37.

Green, L. W. (2006). Public health asks of systems science: To advance our evidence-based practice, can you help us get more practice-based evidence? *American Journal of Public Health, 96*(3), 406–409.

Green, L. W. (2008). Making research relevant: If it is an evidence-based practice, where's the practice-based evidence? *Family Practice: The International Journal for Research in Primary Care, 25*(Suppl. 1), i20–i24. doi:10.1093/fampra/cmn055

Hagan, J., & Walden, M. (2015). Development and evaluation of the barriers to nurses' participation in research questionnaire at a large academic pediatric hospital. *Clinical Nursing Research, 26*(2), 157–175.

Hammond, F. M., Barrett, R., Dijkers, M. P., Zanca, J. M., Horn, S. D., Smout, R. J., . . . Dunning, M. R. (2015). Group therapy use and its impact on the outcomes of inpatient rehabilitation after traumatic brain injury: Data from Traumatic Brain Injury-Practice Based Evidence Project. *Archives of Physical Medicine and Rehabilitation, 96*(8 Suppl.), S282–S292.

Horn, S. D. (1999). Clinical practice improvement: A data-driven methodology for improving patient care. *Journal of Clinical Outcomes Management, 6*(3), 26–32.

Horn, S. D., & Gassaway, J. (2007). Practice-based evidence study design for comparative effectiveness research. *Medical Care, 45*(10 Suppl. 2), S50–S57.

Horn, S. D., & Gassaway, J. (2010). Practice based evidence: Incorporating clinical heterogeneity and patient-reported outcomes for comparative effectiveness research. *Medical Care, 48*(6 Suppl.), S17–S22.

Horn, S. D., Gassaway, J., Pentz, L., & James, R. (2010). Practice-based evidence for clinical practice improvement: An alternative study design for evidence-based medicine. In E. J. S. Hovenga, M. R. Kidd, S. Garde, & L. C. C. Hullin (Eds.), *Health informatics* (pp. 446–460). Amsterdam, The Netherlands: IOS Press.

Institute of Medicine Committee on Quality of Health Care in America. (2001). *Crossing the quality chasm: A new health system for the 21st century.* Washington, DC: National Academies Press.

Issel, L. M. (2016). Health program planning and evaluation: What nurse scholars need to know. In J. R. Bloch, M. R. Courtney, & M. L. Clark (Eds.), *Practice-based clinical inquiry in nursing for DNP and PhD research: Looking beyond traditional methods* (pp. 3–20). New York, NY: Springer Publishing.

Karnick, P. M. (2016). Evidence based practice and nursing theory. *Nursing Science Quarterly, 29*(4), 283–284.

Kolcaba, K. (2003). *Comfort theory and practice: A vision for holistic healthcare and research.* New York, NY: Springer Publishing.

Kuhn, T., & Jackson, M. M. (2008). Accomplishing knowledge: A framework for investigating knowing in organizations. *Management Communication Quarterly, 21*(4), 454–485.

Larson, S. M. (2008). Practice-based evidence of the beneficial impact of positron emission tomography in clinical oncology. *Journal of Clinical Oncology, 26*(3), 2083–2084.

Leeman, J., & Sandelowski, M. (2012). Practice-based evidence and qualitative inquiry. *Journal of Nursing Scholarship, 44*(2), 171–179.

Lin, G. Y., Lin, Y. K., Lee, J. T., Lee, M. S., Lin, C. C., Tsai, C. K., . . . Yang, F. C. (2016). Prevalence of restless legs syndrome in migraine patients with and without aura: A cross-sectional, case-controlled study. *Journal of Headache and Pain, 17*(1), 97. doi:10.1186/s10194-016-0691-0

Linder, L. A., Gerdy, C., Abouzelof, R., & Wilson, A. (2017). Using practice-based evidence to improve supportive care practices to reduce central line-associated bloodstream infections in a pediatric oncology unit. *Journal of Pediatric Oncology Nursing, 34*(3), 185–195.

Long, M. T., & Fox, C. S. (2016). The Framingham heart study—67 years of discovery in metabolic disease. *Nature Reviews Endocrinology, 12*(3), 177–183.

Longino, H. (2002). *The fate of knowledge*. Princeton, NJ: Princeton University Press.

Magyary, D., Whitney, J. D., & Brown, M. A. (2006). Advancing practice inquiry: Research foundations of the practice doctorate in nursing. *Nursing Outlook, 54*(3), 139–151.

McDonald, P. W., & Viehbeck, S. (2007). From evidence-based practice making to practice-based evidence making: Creating communities of (research) and practice. *Health Promotion Practice, 8*(2), 140–144.

Nicholson, J., Hinden. B. R., Biebel, K., Henry, A. D., & Katz-Leavy, J. (2007). A qualitative study of programs for parents with serious mental illness and their children: Building practice-based evidence. *Journal of Behavioral Health Services & Research, 34*(4), 395–413.

Polit, D. F., & Beck, C. T. (2017). *Nursing research: Generating and assessing evidence for nursing practice* (10th ed.). Philadelphia, PA: Wolters Kluwer Health.

Potempa, K. M., Redman, R. W., & Anderson, C. A. (2008). Capacity for the advancement of nursing science: Issues and challenges. *Journal of Professional Nursing, 24*(6), 329–336.

Reed, P. G., & Rishel, C. J. (2015). Epistemic injustice and nurse moral distress. *Nursing Science Quarterly, 28*, 241–244.

Rycroft-Malone, J., Seers, K., Titchen, A., Harvey, G., Kitson, A., & McCormack, B. (2004). What counts as evidence in evidence-based practice? *Journal of Advanced Nursing, 47*(1), 81–90.

Sackett, D. L., Rosenberg, W. M., Gray, J. A., Haynes, R. B., & Richardson, W. S. (1996). Evidence based medicine: What it is and what it isn't. *British Medical Journal, 312*, 71–72.

Salmon, P., & Young, B. (2013). The validity of education and guidance for clinical communication in cancer care: Evidence-based practice will depend on practice-based evidence. *Patient Education and Counseling, 90*, 193–199.

Scala, E., Price, C., & Day, J. (2016). An integrative review of engaging clinical nurses in nursing research. *Journal of Nursing Scholarship, 48*(4), 423–430.

Sidani, S., Doran, D. M., & Mitchell, P. H. (2004). A theory-driven approach to evaluating quality of nursing care. *Journal of Nursing Scholarship, 36*(1), 60–65.

Siebens, H. C., Sharkey, P., Aronow, H. U., Deutscher, D., Roberts, P., Munin, M. C., . . . Horn, S. D. (2016). Variation in rehabilitation treatment patterns for hip fracture treated with arthroplasty. *Physical Medicine & Rehabilitation, 8*(3), 191–207.

Song, M., Hu, F. B., Wu, K., Must, A., Chan, A. T., Willett, W. C., & Giovannucci, E. L. (2016). Trajectory of body shape in early and middle life and all cause and cause specific mortality: Results from two prospective US cohort studies. *British Medical Journal, 353*, i2195. doi:10.1136/bmj.i2195

Staffileno, B. A., Murphy, M. P., & Carlson, E. (2017). Determinants for effective collaboration among DNP- and PhD-prepared faculty. *Nursing Outlook, 65,* 94–102.

Taylor, M. V., Priefer, B. A., & Alt-White, A. C. (2016). Evidence-based practice: Embracing integration. *Nursing Outlook, 64*(6), 575–582.

Udlis, K. A., & Manucuso, J. M. (2015). Perceptions of the role of the doctor of nursing practice-prepared nurse: Clarity or confusion. *Journal of Professional Nursing, 31*(4), 274–283.

Westfall, J. M., Mold, J., & Fagnan, L. (2007). Practice-based research—"Blue Highways" on the NIH Roadmap. *Journal of the American Medical Association, 297*(4), 403–406.

Westra, B. L., Sylvia, M., Weinfurter, E. F., Pruinelli, L., Park, J. I., Dodd, D., . . . Delaney, C. W. (2016). Big data science: A literature review of nursing research exemplars. *Nursing Outlook.* Advance online publication. doi:10.1016/j.outlook .2016.11.021

Zanca, J. M., Natale, A., Labarbera, J., Schroeder, S. T., Gassaway, J., & Backus, D. (2011). Group physical therapy during inpatient rehabilitation for acute spinal cord injury: Findings from the SCIRehab Study. *Physical Therapy, 91*(12), 1877–1891.

Zimmerman, K., Domb, A., Brewer, B. B., & Johnson, R. (2011). Brushing away ventilator-associated pneumonia. *Nursing 2011 Critical Care, 6*(4), 7–11.

12

Interlude IV: *Community-Based Nursing Praxis as a Catalyst for Generating Knowledge*

Cathleen Michaels

Nurses walk many paths in practice that can generate knowledge for the discipline. One path is community. Nurses increasingly are practicing in the community, moving beyond the walls of hospitals and clinics to enhance the health of individuals, families, and other groups in places where people live, work, play, and pray. This chapter focuses on community-based practice, including my own work, as a context for generating nursing knowledge. I also draw from classic references and a philosophy of community praxis to describe how community is a natural context where nurses and community members partner to foster health and health-related knowledge for human welfare.

Much of the knowledge that informs the community-based nurse as guide and coach is embedded in the interactions between nurses, community members and community as a whole. Nursing practice in community with individuals or groups can also be a catalyst for community member knowledge production. Paulo Freire (1970), an internationally renowned educational progressive, advocated knowledge production by ordinary people to identify and resolve problems in everyday life. Nurses' and community members' knowledge production creates opportunity to integrate knowledge for the purpose of working together toward health-related goals.

PERSPECTIVES ON COMMUNITY

Community may be defined geographically or relationally. An example of a community defined geographically is the population of a city with defined boundaries. An example of a community defined relationally is a group of people with chronic obstructive pulmonary disease (COPD) living in close proximity but not necessarily in the same town who meet monthly to discuss approaches to self-managing COPD. With either definition, the essential characteristic of community is a shared identity and interaction between community members (Israel, Checkoway, Schulz, & Zimmerman, 1994; Wilkinson, 1991).

Although the geographical definition prevails in health care, other perspectives about community are helpful for nurses to maintain while working with a community. These perspectives alert nurses to characteristics and resources within a community to draw from in facilitating community-based projects and interventions. In particular, McKnight (1992) provided a perspective about the potential of community, viewing community in terms of its members' assets for working together to solve problems. McKnight (1992) drew from ideas by Alexis de Tocqueville, the French count who visited the United States in 1831 and observed something new among the American citizens:

> First, they were groups of citizens who decided they had the power to decide what was a problem. Second, they decided they had the power to decide how to solve the problem. Third, they often decided that they would themselves become the key actors in implementing the solution. (pp. 57–58)

A community *can-do* spirit reflects a readiness the nurse can build on in working toward health goals for individuals within a community or the community as a whole.

ASSESSING INFLUENCES ON COMMUNITY CAPACITY FOR HEALTH

Nurses are accustomed to describing health in terms of individuals, yet we are also aware that individuals are embedded in various systems or "influential spheres" (Labonte, 1993), including social, cultural, and physical environments. Labonte (1993) explained that if we overemphasize health at the individual level, our practice will define health as an individual process and disregard the significant influence of small groups (such as family and relational communities), geographic community, larger organizations, and the environment on health. He noted that the small group, such as the relational community, was particularly influential for the interpersonal bonds and social support it can provide.

Without this larger perspective of influential spheres, a nurse, for example, may offer a treatment plan to an individual newly diagnosed with diabetes but disregard how his or her family influences his or her eating habits or disregard the social and economic underpinnings that may limit accessibility to health care services and professional support. *Community capacity* for health, which is the human and material resources needed to make a desired change (Norton, McLeroy, Burdine, Felix, & Dorsey, 2002), is increased by these many spheres of community influence. Successful community-based practice is more likely when the nurse understands the contribution of small and large groups to health and can assess and apply the resources of these spheres.

Power relationships also influence community capacity for health and the success of community-based practice. If power is not shared within the community, community capacity to recognize and respond to health issues decreases. The nurse therefore must foster mutuality with community members. Forces that counteract mutuality include ascribing power to the person with the most education and the most resources, as well as holding differing agendas held by the nurse, researchers, and communities. Mutuality between the nurse and community members is reflected in elements of the relationship regarding who has the power to name the problem, make decisions, and manage resources (Labonte, 1997). Power relationships can be overt, subtle, or covert. For a successful community-based practice, it is essential to analyze and monitor power relationships to establish transparency and sustain mutuality.

COMMUNITY PRAXIS: A PERSPECTIVE UNDERLYING COMMUNITY-BASED PRACTICE

Praxis is the action-oriented process through which knowledge can be generated in the context of community-based practice. While there are many perspectives on praxis presented in the literature, from Aristotle to present philosophers, praxis was a key concept for critical theory and social science that emphasized emancipating people to think independently (Carr & Kemmis, 1986). Newman (1994), among several nurse scholars, provides a useful perspective for nursing praxis, explaining praxis as the integration of theory, research, and practice to facilitate health.

In community praxis, the professional and individual or community participate in linking thought (theory) and action in building knowledge and evaluating its application and outcomes. As elaborated by Freire in his 1970 book *Cultural Action for Freedom* (cited in Carr & Kemmis, 1986), outcomes generated through praxis develop through a back and forth between thought and action without a predetermined end point. Newman's (1994) nursing praxis emphasizes a focus on patterns in the back and forth process between thought and action. Shared theory evolves with the nurse as the empirical expert about health, process, and pattern recognition, and the community-based nurse as guide and coach is embedded in the interactions between nurses, community members and community as a whole expert about details that form the patterns and their associated meanings.

Nursing praxis begins with bringing a nursing theoretical perspective about human beings and health to bear on nursing interactions with individuals and communities in a way that helps people recognize their own health patterns, definitions, and desires for health. In a community-based project, nursing praxis becomes a shared or *community praxis* when community members use knowledge of their own health patterns along with other knowledge sources to participate in health-promoting practices. Evaluations of these practices or actions are used to reform or refine the theoretical perspectives that will inform subsequent action. Knowledge and actions are evaluated by action research methods and then result in two outcomes: (a) expanded awareness about one's health patterns and (b) tangible results of the action on health or health practices. Both outcomes can be transformative in bringing about changes in health perspectives and behaviors.

RESPECTFUL DIALOGUE

According to Freire (1970) and Newman (1994), the foundation for praxis is respectful dialogue in which no one person dominates but power is equitably shared through respect for each individual. Without the authenticity and value for multiple perspectives that underlie respectful dialogue, mutuality cannot emerge. Uneven power relationships or lack of mutuality can limit coparticipation in identifying and naming a problem as well as deciding how to respond to the problem with available resources.

CONSCIENTIZATION

Conscientization is a term coined by Freire (1970) to describe awareness of a process of consciousness raising that must precede action. According to Freire in his 1970 book *Cultural Action for Freedom* (as cited in Carr & Kemmis, 1986), conscientization refers to a "... deepening awareness both of the sociohistorical reality which shapes their [people's] lives and of their capacity to transform that reality" (p. 157). Conscientization is based on an approach to teaching that emphasizes questioning mainstream ideas, beliefs, and practices by understanding deeper meanings and root causes. Freire considered conscientization a necessary first step, essential for people to connect their experiences with their social context and confidently consider action for change. For example, in Freire's (1970) Brazilian community, he educated the people not only to read but also to become aware that the inability to read exacerbated oppression of the poor because literacy was required to vote in public elections.

Likewise, Newman (1994) described a process by which patients could consciously connect their experiences into a pattern of the whole. For example, Newman described a method in which the patient tells his life story, describing person–environment interactions that have been most meaningful in life and health; revealing themes about his health patterns and expressing person–environment themes about his health pattern over time. It is not uncommon for patients to meaningfully interact with their environment to promote health, particularly when chronic illness is present. In community-based practice, then, the nurse values and facilitates community member awareness of patterns that express inherent abilities to take a desired action that influences their health and well-being.

PARTICIPATORY ACTION RESEARCH

Research is an important element behind effective community-based practice. The knowledge generated through community-based practice is part of a cycle of knowledge production that includes research to examine the effectiveness of interventions. *Participatory action research* refers to a philosophy and research methods that place high value on knowing through action-based experience coupled with research methods (Reason, 1994). The action-based approach is organized by a cycle of "planning, acting, observing, and reflecting" (Carr & Kemmis, 1986, p. 162). Community-based practice is enhanced when nurse and community members work together in research endeavors to develop and examine interventions. The degree of community participation influences the effectiveness of the intervention, including the relevance of the knowledge that informs the action and the potential for ownership sustaining the effort. Participatory action research aligns with community praxis in ensuring full participation and meaningful outcomes for the community.

EXAMPLE OF COMMUNITY-BASED PRACTICE WITH A GROUP: THE TUCSON HOLISTIC HEALING INITIATIVE FOR NURSES (THHIN)

My work with the THHIN is an example of community praxis. THHIN was a partnership between the University of Arizona College of Nursing and five original hospital partners that progressed to 10 partners. The purpose of the partnership was to promote the health and well-being of hospital staff nurses by exploring and using holistic modalities and integrated therapies in the workplace. Examples of these modalities included deep breathing techniques, aromatherapy, and music therapy.

The group initially convened, discussed, and decided on its purpose, named itself, and planned four consultations for the first year of the project. The consultations focused on creating healing environments and adopting holistic modalities and integrated therapies for work-based self-care practices. Following each consultation, a planning group, consisting of several representatives from each hospital partner and two nurse faculty members who served as facilitators, met to reflect on and discuss the highlights of each consultation to make the next consultation more effective. Although the group began more like a traditional committee, a relational community developed early in the process based on a common interest in THHIN and frequent interactions. Sustaining this relational community was essential to promoting the healing and health of staff nurses. Therefore, "theory" in the form of knowledge about how to sustain this community was critical to the health goals.

In particular, knowledge was generated within the THHIN group regarding approaches to building community capacity and *social capital*, that is, the interpersonal bonds between community members and bridges between hospitals. For example, at the start of THHIN, community capacity was low, indicating a need for more interactions to build social capital (Kreuter & Lezin, 2002). Knowledge from community feedback led to important changes to sustain the community. For example, feedback was translated into decisions to modify the consultations: Community members decided to transform the meetings into "consultations" with fewer meetings but meetings scheduled over breakfast so that all could attend—staff, each hospital champion, and their respective chief nursing officers. Meeting every 2 weeks for a month and then monthly resulted in a rapid increase in social capital as well as an increase in community capacity as human and other resources were mobilized to showcase the consultations. Similar processes of community praxis could be considered in other community-based partnerships.

A STORY ABOUT EVOLVING THEORETICAL CONCEPTS THROUGH COMMUNITY-BASED PRACTICE WITH INDIVIDUALS

My community-based practice provides rich data about partnering with individuals and groups to promote health. Reflections on these experiences from my praxis perspective, along with knowledge about community, helped me generate theoretical concepts out of my practice.

My initial community-based work was with hospitalized individuals. As I spoke to them about being able to support them in the community, I felt uncertain about whether I would be welcomed into their homes after discharge. In general, people feel vulnerable and in need of help when hospitalized but not necessarily so when they are in community. Moreover, I realized that their homes were not professional turf. Nevertheless, I suggested continuing my support beyond the hospital walls. I introduced myself and said that I would like to offer my support to help with any health concerns. When asked about what kind of help I meant, I offered detailed examples based on the nature of their health. One day, a hospital person characterized my offer of help to her friend by explaining that the hospital had sent her a *partner.* In describing the beginning relationship between the nurse and the patient then, I would say that a conversation had initiated relationship, the health issues and potential support established context for the relationship, and labeling the relationship as *partnership* moved the relationship beyond the hospital walls into the community.

During my visits in the community, I endeavored to deepen the relationships between myself and individuals by, primarily, listening. I listened to them tell stories about their illness experience, their sense of cause and consequence, and their perspectives about what makes them feel better and worse. My support of their understanding of illness and their acceptance of my questions and comments about their illness cocreated our relationship. As time progressed, we increased our sense of self in the relationship, sharing knowledge and acting together as partners to promote health.

THEORETICAL CONCEPTS FROM PRACTICE

From reflections on my community-based practice, I identified key concepts, particularly as they illuminated how I engaged and sustained relationships with patients in the community. This interest in "how" and asking "how" questions underlies and generates theoretical thinking in and about practice.

The first concept to emerge in my theorizing was *connectedness.* I selected the concept of connectedness to refer to the *nature* of my relationships as individuals progressed from discussing hospital discharge to community. The initial connectedness varied and ranged from simply being invited into the home to being heartily welcomed with a thoughtfully planned tea party, as demonstrated by Helen, a

75-year-old widow who lived alone in a senior community. My initial visit with Helen took place at her home since she had been seen only in the emergency room, not the hospital. For my second home visit, Helen set up a tea table for two. She placed a white sheet over her coffee table and used her meager resources to provide tea and cake. This concept of connectedness represents a genuine, authentic relationship between myself and another person, represented by Helen's heartfelt actions in preparing the tea party for us to enjoy together. Thus, I used connectedness—as a transferable concept—to conceptually frame my work with other individuals in the community.

The second concept I identified was *partnership* as inspired by Helen's characterization of my role with individuals in the community. I defined this concept as a *process*, referring to how the two of us worked together as partners toward health-related goals. Our partnership was formed as we explicitly agreed to work together.

The third concept that I adopted was *mutual endeavor*. I described this concept in terms of the *content* of our relationship, which focused on our mutual goal of finding ways to enhance the individual's health situation. Without mutual agreement on the goal, a relationship is one sided and therefore not fully functional and unable to meet its potential.

The fourth concept I identified from my practice was *mutual benefit*. This concept reflects an *outcome* of the process. Most notably, the individual benefits from improved health outcomes as well as from other positive experiences in interactions with the nurse. The nurse may also benefit through the communication and emotional connections with another human being, as well as through the learning that occurs in interacting and caring for another. Without acknowledging these positive experiences for the nurse, the nurse's authenticity in knowledge and action cannot be fully established as true and genuine.

SCOTTY: AN EXAMPLE OF THE LINK BETWEEN ACTION AND THEORY

When I consider the theoretical concepts, particularly *mutual benefit*, that have emerged from my community-based practice, I think of my work with Scotty. Scotty was a 78-year-old community member and patient. He was an intriguing person—independent and living alone with no social support other than talking to the clerk at the Walgreen's across the street from his residence and who kept $10,000 in a jar in the refrigerator in case he "had to leave town quickly." Healthwise, he had a difficult time believing in physiology as dynamic and influenced by his health practices, as evidenced by his belief that a "good" blood pressure would be one where the systolic and diastolic values should always be the same numbers. Scotty confided that he was going to buy cedar berries and stop taking his oral antiglycemic agent. His evidence for making this decision was a physician letter to the editor in a local newspaper that declared diabetes can be cured with cedar berries.

While I had high personal value for Scotty's autonomy and self-determination, I also knew that unless he altered his health practices, Scotty could likely end up hospitalized again with hyperosmolar coma secondary to hyperglycemia. To acknowledge both of my perspectives, I affirmed to Scotty that it was his decision whether or not he took his medication or cedar berries, but I also suggested that he learn to monitor his blood glucose to know how his diabetes was responding. I was working from my belief in Scotty's inner strengths and from the idea that by helping Scotty learn more about his health patterns, he would make better informed decisions about his health practices related to his diabetes.

Scotty did learn to check his blood sugar using a glucometer. He systematically checked his blood sugar before and after meals, reflecting on the results from different foods he ate and his various activities such as walking around the block. After 3 months of measuring his blood sugar and recording the results, Scotty told me he decided to continue taking his diabetic medications because he did not want to "rock the boat." I breathed a sigh of relief because he had reflected and then chosen to continue this important self-management practice.

In reflecting on my own practice, I realized that my values for autonomy and self-determination coupled with my expert knowledge about diabetes and interpersonal relationships helped me create an effective glucose monitoring feedback system with Scotty. Through our *partnership*, which was buttressed by our *connectedness*, Scotty came to a better understanding of the influences and outcomes of glycemic control, which enabled and motivated him to decide to continue his medications. I approached our work as a *mutual endeavor*, accounting for both his values and mine in the interactions. The outcome was one of *mutual benefit* in that Scotty chose a health practice that would benefit him, and I gained both personal fulfillment and professional knowledge for my work in the community. I also confirmed through another source that there is evidence that cedar berries lower blood sugar. For me, this represented Scotty's own self-determination and wisdom that he brought to his own health care, which made us truly partners in his health care.

Research guided by a framework of these concepts might obtain empirical support for relationships between concepts. It is conceivable that the three concepts—connectedness, partnership, and mutual endeavor—together contribute significantly to mutual benefit for the nurse and care-recipient well-being. Such a theory could truly reflect holistic nursing practice that addresses both participants in the health care relationship.

CONCLUSIONS: A COMMUNITY PRAXIS APPROACH TO PRACTICE AND KNOWLEDGE

Health-related action and knowledge production in community-based practice occurs through partnership of the nurse, community members, and community as a whole. It is important for the nurse to understand a community's inherent strengths and challenges, accounting for community identity and diversity, and assessing power relationships and other factors that influence community capacity for health.

Community praxis is a perspective useful to nurses who engage a community in the coproduction of knowledge though community-based practice. The goals of community-based nursing practice are achieved by engaging the community in addressing a given health concern by mutually deciding what the problem is, what to do about it, and how to know if the action is successful. *Community praxis* provides a perspective of partnering with individuals in the community to support the inherent strengths of the members and community as a whole, while helping to free participants from social constraints and resolve problems to enhance in their health and well-being.

My practice with communities, like THHIN and with community members like Scotty and Helen highlight my praxis perspective and value for partnership. Reflections on my practice have helped me develop theoretical ideas about how nurses and patients can join together to integrate knowledge for action. I identified four positively-related concepts that can be organized into a framework to guide theory development and community-based practice. Unique to this framework is the integration of theory and action in proposing links among partnership, connectedness, and mutual endeavor for the mutual benefit of patients and nurses.

SUMMARY POINTS

1. Community is a natural context where nurses and community members partner to foster health and health-related knowledge for human welfare.

2. Community-based nursing practice from a praxis perspective is a process of championing community strengths and knowledge along with nursing expertise and knowledge in sustaining partnerships that facilitate health.

3. A reflective, praxis approach to community nursing practice can generate theoretical concepts that may be organized into a framework to help guide interactions that benefit the well-being of both the nurse and the care recipient.

 QUESTIONS FOR REFLECTION

1. How would you evaluate the usefulness of the community praxis perspective presented here in your own work with patients?

2. How might you use the partnership approach to develop ideas for knowledge or theory development in your area of research?

3. What ideas do you have about other approaches to linking theory and practice that might extend or differ from the ideas presented in this chapter?

4. From your own experiences, what theoretical concepts might you identify that could be helpful in building theory to address the same health problem across different patients?

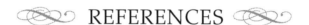 REFERENCES

Carr, W., & Kemmis, S. (1986). *Becoming critical: Education, knowledge and action research.* London, England: The Falmer Press.

Freire, P. (1970). *Pedagogy of the oppressed.* New York, NY: The Seabury Press.

Israel, B. A., Checkoway, B., Schulz, A., & Zimmerman, M. (1994). Health education and community empowerment: Conceptualizing and measuring perceptions of individual, organizational, and community control. *Health Education Quarterly, 21,* 149–170.

Kreuter, M. W., & Lezin, N. (2002). Social capital theory: Implications for community-based health promotion. In R. J. DiClemente, R. A. Crosby, & M. C. Kegler (Eds.), *Emerging theories in health promotion, practice and research* (pp. 228–254). San Francisco, CA: Jossey-Bass.

Labonte, R. (1993). The empowerment holosphere. In R. Labonte (Ed.), *Health promotion and empowerment: Practice frameworks* (Issues in Health Promotion Series Monograph, HP-10–0102, pp. 59–89). Toronto, ON, Canada: Centre for Health Promotion, University of Toronto and ParticipACTION.

Labonte, R. (1997). Community, community development and the forming of authentic partnerships: Some critical reflections. In M. Minkler (Ed.), *Community organization and community building for health* (pp. 82–96). New Brunswick, NJ: Rutgers University Press.

McKnight, J. L. (1992). Redefining community. *Social Policy, 23*(2), 56–62.

Newman, M. (1994). *Health as expanding consciousness* (2nd ed.). New York, NY: National League for Nursing Press.

Norton, B. L., McLeroy, K. R., Burdine, J. N., Felix, M. R. J., & Dorsey, A. M. (2002). Community capacity. In R. J. DiClemente, R. A. Crosby, & M. C. Kegler (Eds.), *Emerging theories in health promotion, practice and research* (pp. 194–227). San Francisco, CA: Jossey-Bass.

Reason, P. (1994). Three approaches to participative inquiry. In N. K. Denzin & Y. S. Lincoln (Eds.), *Handbook of qualitative research* (pp. 324–339). Thousand Oaks, CA: Sage.

Wilkinson, K. (1991). *The community in rural America*. Westport, CN: Greenwood Press.

13

A Paradigm for the Production of Practice-Based Knowledge: Philosophical and Practical Considerations[1]

Pamela G. Reed

No one owns science. If we wish to make informed choices, we must never forget that science exists because people created it, and it cannot exist separate from the community. Behind all the . . . professional degrees, the idea of science—our long effort to understand nature—and the knowledge that radiates from that search, are part of our shared human heritage.

Ede and Cormack, 2004, p. 420

From composers to scientists, innovation and discovery are highly valued by society and by the innovators themselves. Beethoven, for example, believed so deeply in innovation and individual expression above ritual and tradition that the originality of each of his nine symphonies limited him to composing far fewer symphonies than his predecessors (Grove, 1962). Conner's (2005) compelling account of the history of science reveals the significance of the artisans—people who worked with their hands—in the development of knowledge and the Scientific Revolution. The artisans transformed know-how into knowledge through the daily practices of their work, which involved ongoing experimentation, intervention, and the use of instruments.

1. Adapted from P. G. Reed and L. A. Lawrence. (2008). A paradigm for the production of practice-based knowledge. *Journal of Nursing Management, 16*, 422–432. Copyright © Blackwell Publishers Ltd. Reprinted with permission by John Wiley and Sons.

The birth of modern science occurred, Conner (2005) explains, when the intellectual elite engaged in "knowledge robbery," appropriating artisans' knowledge and then systematizing it. The artisans' "latent contribution to science" did not reap recognition as learned individuals, but it significantly advanced knowledge during the Middle Ages. Artisans' work also brought forth a method of knowledge production that connected the scientist to nature rather than ancient authority.

The contributions of practicing nurses to the well-being of patients and the viability of health care systems are indisputable. Like the artisans of the past, practicing nurses today are not recognized for their production of knowledge. In fact, within our current paradigm of knowledge development, most nurses are socialized into being users, not producers, of knowledge. This chapter explores issues and trends surrounding knowledge production in nursing and proposes a paradigm of knowledge development to promote nursing knowledge production among practicing nurses. *Nursing knowledge* refers to knowledge warranted as useful and significant to nurses and patients in understanding and facilitating human health processes.

THE KNOWLEDGE DISTINCTION IN A PROFESSION

One important characteristic of a profession is that its practice is accompanied by a dynamic system of knowledge development. The persons who develop knowledge are most frequently called scientists, scholars, and researchers, but generally not practitioners. Nursing distinguishes between the knowledge producers and the knowledge users; those designated as the knowledge producers typically are educated in research-based rather than in practice-based doctoral programs. This knowledge distinction within a discipline can weaken capacity for knowledge production while also diminishing practitioners' jurisdiction over their practice (Abbott, 1988; Reed, 2016; Urban, 2013).

MARGINALIZING NURSING PRACTICE KNOWLEDGE

It is better to do than to judge, to produce than to evaluate, to create than to criticize, to invent than to classify copies. Playing is better than blowing the referee's whistle.

Serres, 1995, p. 128

For all they do and know, practitioners remain an untapped dimension of knowledge development in our discipline. The American Association of Colleges of Nursing (AACN) identified those with research doctorates to be the knowledge producers of the discipline, who then transmit knowledge to practicing nurses who are expected to "use and evaluate, but not conduct, research" (AACN, 2004). The academy (AACN, 2015) has since clarified its position further, viewing doctors of nursing practice (DNPs) as well as PhDs as generators of knowledge, though not by using rigorous research. Nevertheless, practitioners are already knowledge producers in a most basic and elegant manner—they are confronted with new situations every time a patient walks through the door and are capable of integrating new information to explain how these situations are best dealt with (Lum, 2002). Nursing is in need of more nurses who can expand, not just evaluate, its knowledge base.

Segregating knowledge users from knowledge producers promotes exclusivity in knowledge generation where the few generate knowledge for the many. Current statistics by the U.S. National Sample Survey of Registered Nurses (NSSRN) indicate that 1% of nurses are developing knowledge for the other 99% of nurses (U.S. Department of Health and Human Services and Health Resources and Services Administration, 2010). This segregation harkens memories of the media and the public questioning the nurse's right to engage in independent research and publication "without the imprimatur of a physician" (Downs, 1991, p. 195).

Epistemological decisions about who are the legitimate knowers and knowledge producers in nursing have sociopolitical implications for practice (Bart, 2000). Clinicians who are perceived as lacking the ability to produce knowledge for their practice are more vulnerable to falling under the jurisdiction of other health care professionals. Because the discipline has not shaken loose an operative ontology of "physician's orders," tens of thousands of nurses still follow physicians' orders and, in many states, they follow physician assistants' orders. It is inconsistent with professional practice that nursing practices are dependent on physicians' orders to implement nursing care, such as ambulating or turning patients, entering consults to other disciplines, and ordering durable equipment for end-of-life care. Nurses have not fully enacted or transferred the scope and substance of their knowledge to practice.

Sociologist Andrew Abbott (1988) studied the system of professions and determined that abstract knowledge is a major element in a profession's level of jurisdiction or control over practice. He explained that professions have varying forms of jurisdiction over their practice: Some professions share jurisdiction over practice with each other, as with attorneys and certified public accountants; some have an advisory relationship, such as that between clergy and medicine; other professions have control over cognitive knowledge but not over their practice such as that between psychotherapists and psychiatrists. Abbott (1988) used nursing as the exemplar of the most limited form of jurisdiction over one's practice, which he called "subordination."

Abbott (1988) explained that a profession's jurisdiction over practice depends in large part on the educational level of the profession. However, perhaps more importantly, he found that level of jurisdiction was related to the presence of abstract thinking or theories used in practice. Mechanics, for example, are not professionals per se, but if they possessed the abstract knowledge of an engineer to link their observations and technical prowess to theoretical explanations, they could be. The same goes for practicing nurses and their knowledge. Jurisdiction and autonomy are difficult to achieve without the requisite knowledge and knowledge-building skills, a critical process sometimes overlooked in the familiar path from novice to expert.

BLACK-BOXING NURSING PRACTICE KNOWLEDGE

The discipline of nursing grew out of a public demand for knowledgeable caregivers (Fagin, 2000), and nursing is recognized as the profession of caregiving. However, nurses' caregiving knowledge has been "black-boxed"—a metaphor used by Latour (1999) to indicate that a work or a technology "has been made invisible by its own success" (p. 304). Black-boxing occurs when a complexity of elements act as one. It is a metaphor symbolizing the closing off of continued interest, appreciation, and inquiry into a dynamic source of scientific knowledge and rendering it as an "opaque object of fact" (Sturman, 2006, p. 182).

Black-boxing occurs in nursing when the complexity of behaviors and ideas that come together in nurses' acts of caregiving are invisible and not well understood or fully appreciated; however, paradoxically, black-boxed knowledge is considered credible and too costly to understand or replace. Caregiving becomes transparent, a taken-for-granted yet integral reality of health care. Furthermore, what is black-boxed is considered compact and portable. The professional practice of cross-coverage and use of traveling nurses are visible examples of black-boxing nurses' caregiving knowledge and skills within nursing practice. Nurses are imported to practice within the context of a new unit. In so doing, knowledge is separated from the context of its discovery (Latour & Woolgar, 1986). Further, to the extent that other health care professions do not recognize the knowledge potential and knowledge produced in the context of caregiving, but benefit from it, "knowledge robbery" occurs—similar to that which occurred among 16th-century artisans. As a result, nurses may try to legitimize their practices only by moral or technical approaches to health care rather than by a scientific understanding of their work (Nelson & Gordon, 2006).

KNOWLEDGE PRODUCTION CAUGHT BETWEEN TWO PARADIGMS OF PRACTICE

This deficit in nursing knowledge and nursing-ordered practices has created a vacuum, which two paradigms of practice knowledge, "evidence-based" and "expert intuitive-practitioner" (Purkis & Bjornsdottir, 2006), have rushed in to fill. Each paradigm offers important perspectives for nursing practice but is insufficient for supporting nurse clinicians as knowledge workers.

Evidence-based practice is usually broad enough to include the clinician's judgment and patient preferences and values, along with empirical evidence on clinical effectiveness of a treatment. However, it emphasizes knowledge from the scientist's perspective and packaged ahead of time for use, irrespective of the particular context and current contingencies. Evidence-based practice seeks to access knowledge, not to develop knowledge; it does not seek to answer questions about what is actually wrong with a patient and about the underlying mechanisms of the patient's problem and potential solutions (see Fineout-Overholt, Melnyk, & Schultz, 2005; Roberts & Yeager, 2004). To be an empowered professional with jurisdiction over practice, nurses need to be able to participate in knowledge production.

The *intuitive-expert paradigm* of nursing practice originated with Benner's (1984) *From Novice to Expert* and depicts the nurse as an "intuitive knower" and "primary judge" of the legitimacy of the nurse's clinical knowledge (Purkis & Bjornsdottir, 2006, p. 250). This model is practitioner centered with a focus on the present context. It lacks the advantage of an external perspective and critique to inform nurses' judgments about what is "emancipating, good, healthful, and other value-laden concepts" that influence nursing judgment (Reed, 2006). In addition, experience and expert-based sources of knowledge such as craft knowledge, know-how, or tacit knowledge represent the mystery and complexity of how professional practitioners think (Montgomery, 2006); however, equating these types of knowledge with nurses' practice knowledge and then rendering them ineffable stifles nursing's ability both to develop knowledge in and for practice and to marshal evidence of the effectiveness of nursing knowledge, judgment, and skill.

Related to this intuitive-expert model is what Nelson and Gordon (2006) describe as a "narrowed caring discourse," which minimizes recognition of the technical, scientific, and physical practices involved in providing health care and contributes to a simplistic view of nursing care and nursing knowledge by the public and politicians. This "new Cartesianism" focuses on the interpersonal relationship and emotional connection while ignoring the "skills and complexity of body work" (p. 4). They criticize nurses and nursing organizations' heavy emphasis on nurses' virtues rather than on observable, knowledge-based contributions; this "virtue script" is impossible to enact satisfactorily in a hierarchical health care system where it instead "trivializes" nurses' complexity and competencies.

Each of these practice models alone is inadequate in guiding knowledge development for a discipline as complex and dynamic as nursing. But a pluralistic paradigm that brings together evidence-based and caring-focused practice perspectives may be used to facilitate knowledge production among practicing nurses and in so doing increase the autonomy and effectiveness of nursing practice.

A PARADIGM FOR PRACTICE-BASED KNOWLEDGE

Philosophers and scientists are embracing a pluralistic view of science and knowledge development that integrates practice-based knowledge and scientific knowing, and, as such, may be used to facilitate greater participation of practicing nurses in knowledge development. This pluralistic view is found in contemporary philosophies including Longino's (2002) philosophy of *critical contextual empiricism*, Reed's (1995, 2011) *intermodern* philosophy (formerly called neomodernism (2006), and Gibbons et al.'s (1994) *Mode 2 Knowledge Production* (also see Delanty, 2001). In this mode, knowledge production is characterized by its heterogeneity (bringing together diverse skills and experiences to address a problem), reflexivity (involving reflection on values and perspectives of all actors involved), and transdisciplinarity (where knowledge is context sensitive and problem oriented and may transcend traditional disciplinary boundaries, such as those between the university and health care center).

This expanded view of knowledge paves the way for knowledge production in clinical practice settings and provides for a more distinct role for practice viewed as a generative source, if not a prerequisite, to developing nursing knowledge and theory (Reed, 1995). A pluralistic view of nursing knowledge still values the empirical and the theoretical, and the traditional role of critique and consensus in establishing truths, but what qualifies as empirical has gone beyond empiricism to include qualitative as well as quantitative data, stories, and words, as well as measures and numbers. This view also takes into account the influences on knowledge development of such social factors of science as the method and context of inquiry (clinical or laboratory, for example), values and beliefs of the knowledge producer, and the multiple ways of knowing including scientific, ethical, and sociopolitical. Andrew Pickering (1995) captured this new view of knowledge production in a way quite applicable to clinical practice with his description of science as a "mangle" of social, technical, conceptual, political, and personal practices.

The purpose in pluralism is not to remedy inadequacies in any one method of knowledge production alone through some relativist view or to synthesize or resolve paradoxes but to construct places that can sustain the conversation to explore and develop a variety of approaches for their value in building knowledge and solving problems. "Paradoxical, creative thinking, tempered by tolerance for ambiguity is essential in nursing science practice and it . . . distinguishes the clinical expert in nursing science from the rigid and rule-bound procedural technician in nursing" (Rawnsley, 2000, p. 232).

THEORY: A TOOL OF KNOWLEDGE DEVELOPMENT

The 21st-century and post-postmodern or intermodern perspectives (Reed, 1995, 2011) have ushered in new thinking about nursing theory consistent with the paradigm of practice-based knowledge presented previously. Theory as redefined within these new perspectives is a useful tool for practitioners in knowledge development and in achieving the level of abstract knowledge needed to support jurisdiction over practice (Abbott, 1988). Rigid application and preservation of nursing theories understandably have chilled nurses' appreciation for theories' roles in practice. It is not so much that theories are too abstract or difficult to understand as much as they constrain nursing practice and creativity when regarded as an unchangeable voice of authority.

Within this new paradigm of knowledge production, theories are not meant to be applied in a cook-book manner directly to practice but rather to be used, modified, and refined in conjunction with the nurse's creative critical reasoning and interactions with patients. In this way, theory can accommodate the "unforeseeable moments" and reflect an understanding of the way "nursing is lived in practice" (Salas, 2005, p. 22).

The word *theory* is used here to refer to conceptualizations at all levels of abstraction, from broad conceptual frameworks to theories focused on a specific situation (Higgins & Moore, 2000). A theory defined broadly is a dynamic system of concepts that provides an organized perspective, explanation, or probabilistic prediction of an aspect of reality or human experience. This system of concepts also connects us with a larger perspective of the world that cannot be seen from within the immediate context of discovery. Theories are the building blocks of knowledge in a discipline. They provide a degree of effectiveness, dependability, and longevity useful in practice, although every theory is tentative. Theories can move the practitioner beyond the present to facilitate some understanding of "principles, processes and mechanisms that produce or underlie what is present to us" (Longino, 2002, p. 124). In addition, theories may be transported to other relevant contexts for use, beyond the one where they were generated.

Within a pluralistic view of knowledge development, truth is relational, not representational; theories derive their meaning through participation of all of those who share certain practices within a nursing community rather than from correspondence to some fixed indicator of reality (Reed, 2001). Scientific theory does not have to be universal or meet the claim that it will always apply, but it has to stand up to criteria and criticism by a relevant community, such as a certain community of patients or caregivers. Longino (2002) explains that this criticism involves showing how the theory's claims have been systematically generated, how they meet certain goals of the community, and then being open to making needed modifications. For example, modifications may be needed in the scope of the theory's claims or in the knowledge production or research process itself.

The nature of nursing—involving daily encounters with the complexity, uniqueness, and the unpredictability of human beings' health needs—requires that nurses think theoretically and speak of their knowledge. Nurses look for patterns, make connections, posit possible explanations about their observations, and test out and revise their ideas as the situation changes. Nurses are encouraged to question prevailing paradigms of knowledge development that may inhibit their own creative thinking (Meleis & Im, 1999).

The use of theory-based knowledge distinguishes the technical from the professional. Technical workers use what is at hand with less thought about reflecting on their own theories or importing other ideas to explain why things work. This at-handness is the realm of the practical, the immediate, and the unmediated. However, professional workers, members of a discipline, import materials, theories, skills, and technology from elsewhere to enhance their work (Ingraham, 1998).

KNOWLEDGE PRODUCTION IN PRACTICE: STRATEGIES AND INNOVATIONS

Integration of knowledge development into practice opens up opportunities for practicing nurses to participate actively and creatively in addressing vexing health care problems. The following are examples of conceptual, practical, and technological innovations in knowledge production to improve patient care: Discovering how to use the theoretical concepts of "expanding consciousness" to facilitate patient well-being at the end of life (Barron, 2005) and "pattern recognition" to enhance the well-being of women with multiple sclerosis (Neill, 2005); developing a new professional development model that reduces cost and increases nurses' work effectiveness and satisfaction (Bournes & Ferguson-Paré, 2007); adapting an existing evidence-based oral care program for the needs of a specific nursing unit to decrease non-ventilator–associated pneumonia (Federwisch, 2007); or innovating a nursing procedure that hastens healing of a below-the-knee amputation (Dolde, 2007).

The mindful use of theory separates the technical from the professional worker, who seeks knowledge that is not just descriptive but is also explanatory. It is not enough to know *that* an intervention works; it is important to know why and how it works (Lum, 2002). Theoretical thinking provides the means to better understand and judge the evidence for nursing interventions. Practitioners already possess cognitive and experiential skills to engage in theoretical thinking (Marrs & Lowry, 2006). The following are a few of the strategies to support theoretical thinking and knowledge development in practice.

CLINICAL CONCEPTUAL FRAMEWORKS

Conceptual frameworks are an effective first step in theorizing—that is, in transforming observations, interactions, and other data into a form of theory. Knowledge development among practicing nurses depends on their abilities to clearly articulate their operative frameworks and to develop their personal theories. Conceptual frameworks, which are broader in scope and have less detail, are often easier to work with initially when beginning to organize ideas about some phenomenon. Conceptual frameworks are less specific than theories; they simplify structures, highlight the phenomena of interest, and provide a transportable model of some aspect of interest to the practitioner as knowledge producer (Lenoir, 1997). Conceptual frameworks facilitate knowledge production by mapping out the general territory of inquiry, suggesting questions to be asked and observations to be made.

Clinical conceptual frameworks may resemble extant nursing theories or they may be unique to the practitioner and the concepts relevant in practice. Frameworks are flexible conceptual innovations. They may point to general laws of human functioning, or they may portray a process of change or well-being that is relevant to the practice situation at hand. Nurses may use conceptual frameworks to build knowledge with other professionals or with patients, for example, by unmasking misconceptions, positing radically different perspectives of health processes, and helping patients to clarify their experiences and illuminate new meanings of health (Seigfried, 1996).

Philosophers of science suggest that conceptual models or frameworks facilitate dialogue between research and theory because models are at the same time models of observed phenomena and models of theory (Lenoir, 1997). The practitioner can extend knowledge beyond that found in close readings of the canon (the extant conceptual frameworks) and inspire development of bold, new frameworks for deriving hypotheses and practice innovations. In a closed system of knowledge development dominated by traditional scientist views about reality, which assumes that there is a fixed theory or reality independent of mind and language, scientific progress would end once all that there is to discover is discovered (Horgan, 1996). However, the clinical conceptual framework, as part of a dynamic knowledge system, is a mechanism for handling new sources of knowledge brought in through the practitioner's daily interfaces with society. These interfaces create possibilities for new knowledge to emerge that cannot be explained by existing laws. Carrier (2000) called this a process of emergence, where new ideas cannot be explained by existing knowledge. *Caregiving is a gateway to emergent theories for nursing practices.*

PARTNERSHIPS FOR KNOWLEDGE PRODUCTION

Knowledge sharing between clinicians and academics occurs more readily when knowledge is regarded as a gift rather than a commodity, that is, as something to be shared and refined among people committed to understanding and promoting health. Thatchenkery and Chowdhry (2007) describe a process of knowledge management called *appreciative inquiry* that facilitates knowledge generation by accessing knowledge from outside sources. They labeled the specific strategy *appreciative sharing of knowledge* (ASK) that is used to generate and transfer knowledge across systems or organizations.

As universities become more like firms and firms or hospitals become more like universities (Delanty, 2001), institutions may swap strategies to promote knowledge production. For example, hospitals could mandate hours (that are figured into staffing ratios) dedicated to education, sabbaticals, and participation in research conferences for practitioners. Bournes and Ferguson-Paré (2007) described an innovation by which nurses spent 80% of their salaried time in direct patient care and 20% of their time on professional development. Positive outcomes included increased patient and staff satisfaction and nonexistent turnover.

RECOGNIZING THE PRACTITIONER AS CLINICAL SCHOLAR

Clinical scholars participate in both the application of knowledge through practice and in the production of knowledge through inquiry. In addition, the clinical scholar is able to partner with researchers and patients in developing practice-based knowledge. Clinical scholars are skilled at interfacing with various contexts to develop knowledge. They are pivotal in bringing together the objective perspectives of the researcher and the scientist, the subjective views of the patient, and their own patterns of knowing—personal, empirical, ethical, aesthetic, sociopolitical.

Clinical scholars are knowledge managers in sifting, analyzing, and discerning what is important given a diversity of data. However, the data will not yield up theories by themselves. So, clinical scholars are also knowledge producers—linking empirical to the theoretical to explain events and helping patients recognize patterns and meaning in what they are experiencing so they can participate more fully in their own health. The clinical scholar regards knowledge as a process, not a product. The answers are never final because patient contexts and conditions change, and knowledge itself changes. Clinical scholars use theories to enhance their abilities to anticipate change and see the bigger picture.

LOOKING FORWARD: THE *EDGE EFFECT*

New thinking about knowledge production recognizes the synergy in bringing together two systems: the system of knowledge development and the system of practice. This is evident by the prevalence of terms such as *clinical scholar, practitioner/ researcher, scholarly practitioner,* and *scientist–clinician* in the literature and in our conversations. Where practice and research meet creates an *edge effect,* a term used to describe what happens when two ecosystems come together. The renowned cellist Yo-Yo Ma used this term to explain the productive interactions of culturally diverse edges of his life and art (Keller, 2007). The edge effect has the "least density and the greatest variety" (Keller, 2007) and generates new ideas and innovations. Similarly, philosopher Michael Serres (1995) described the interface between systems, such as between science and art, as "the place where things happen." With help from clinical leaders and managers, the practice setting can be a place where innovation and the development of new knowledge can happen.

Having a voice in the underlying ideas and direction of one's practice can be a pivotal element in promoting quality nursing care and in attracting and retaining nurses in the profession. I agree with Anderson (2001), in her commentary on how to achieve a culture of excellence and achievement amid the "challenged" status of nursing: "To surpass the current level . . . stretch the boundary of what is possible, be intolerant of the ordinary, be creative " (p. 209). May this paradigm of practice-based knowledge production become a movement away from the traditional, normal science and into what Kuhn (1962/1996) called "extraordinary science"—a period of ferment and theoretical experimentation in which the practices and concepts of so-called normal science are loosened in ever more radical ways in response to a persistent problem that resists solution within the limits of the prevailing normal science paradigm.

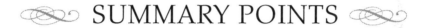

SUMMARY POINTS

1. Knowledge distinctions within a discipline can weaken capacity for knowledge production while also diminishing practitioners' jurisdiction over their practice.

2. There are two paradigms of practice knowledge, evidence-based and intuitive-expert, neither of which alone is adequate for supporting the discipline's knowledge needs.

3. A pluralistic view of knowledge is a paradigm for facilitating knowledge production among practicing nurses.

4. Theory and theoretical thinking are major tools for knowledge development in practice.

5. Strategies can be used to promote innovations in knowledge development for practice.

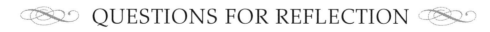

QUESTIONS FOR REFLECTION

1. What do you perceive are some potential benefits of practice-based knowledge production in advancing patient care?

2. What are potential challenges of practice-based knowledge production given the current climate in health care? What are some ways to meet these challenges for the benefit of nursing and patient care?

3. What ideas do you have about potential innovations or strategies in health care settings (your own or in general) that would support your activities as a knowledge producer in practice?

4. What strategies mentioned in this chapter appeal to you in your role as a knowledge producer in nursing (e.g., promoting partnerships, developing a clinical conceptual framework)?

5. Do you think that practice-based knowledge development is important in advancing the voice of nursing in health care?

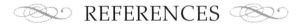 REFERENCES

Abbott, A. (1988). *The system of professions*. Chicago, IL: University of Chicago Press.

American Association of Colleges of Nursing. (2004). *Position statement on the practice doctorate in nursing*. Washington, DC: Author. Retrieved from http://www.aacn nursing.org/Portals/42/News/Position-Statements/DNP.pdf

American Association of Colleges of Nursing. (2015). *The doctor of nursing practice: Current issues and clarifying recommendations*. Washington, DC: Author. Retrieved from http://www.aacnnursing.org/Portals/42/DNP/DNP-Implementation.pdf?ver =2017-08-01-105830-517

Anderson, C. A. (2001). A culture of excellence and achievement. *Nursing Outlook, 49,* 209.

Barron, A. (2005). Suffering, growth and possibility: Health as expanding consciousness in end-of-life care. In C. Picard & D. Jones (Eds.), *Giving voice to what we know* (pp. 43–52). Boston, MA: Jones & Bartlett.

Bart, J. (2000). Feminist theories of knowledge. In J. Bart (Ed.), *Women succeeding in the sciences: Theories and practices across disciplines* (pp. 205–220). West Lafayette, IN: Purdue University Press.

Benner, P. (1984). *From novice to expert*. Menlo Park, CA: Addison-Wesley.

Bournes, D. A., & Ferguson-Paré, M. (2007). Human becoming and 80/20: An innovative professional development model for nurses. *Nursing Science Quarterly, 20,* 237–253.

Carrier, M. (2000). *Science at century's end: Philosophical questions on the progress and limits of science*. Pittsburgh, PA: University of Pittsburgh Press.

Conner, C. D. (2005). *A people's history of science: Miners, midwives, and "low mechanics."* New York, NY: Nation.

Delanty, G. (2001). *Challenging knowledge: The university in the knowledge society*. Philadelphia, PA: Open University Press.

Dolde, K. (2007). Pioneering work in wound care/gastroenterology. *News—Line for Nursing, 8*(40), 4–7.

Downs, F. S. (1991). Informing the media. *Nursing Outlook, 40,* 195.

Ede, A., & Cormack, L. B. (2004). *A history of science in society: From philosophy to utility.* Orchard Park, NY: Broadview Press/Addison-Wesley.

Fagin, C. (2000). *Essays on nursing leadership.* New York, NY: Springer Publishing.

Federwisch, A. (2007). Bright ideas: RNs creating a culture of change. *Nurse Week, 8*(12), 10–11.

Fineout-Overholt, E., Melnyk, B. M., & Schultz, A. (2005). Transforming health care from the inside out: Advancing evidence based practice in the 21st century. *Journal of Professional Nursing, 21,* 335–344.

Gibbons, J., Limoges, C., Nowotny, H., Schwartzman, S., Scot, P., & Trow, M. (1994). *The new production of knowledge: The dynamics of science and research in contemporary societies.* Thousand Oaks, CA: Sage.

Grove, G. (1962). *Beethoven and his nine symphonies.* New York, NY: Dover.

Higgins, P. A., & Moore, M. M. (2000). Levels of theoretical thinking in nursing. *Nursing Outlook, 48,* 179–183.

Horgan, J. (1996). *The end of science.* New York, NY: Addison-Wesley.

Ingraham, C. (1998). *Architecture and the burdens of linearity.* New Haven, NJ: Yale University Press.

Keller, J. (2007). Yo-Yo Ma's edge effect. *Chronicle of Higher Education, 23,* B10–B13.

Kuhn, T. S. (1996). *The structure of scientific revolutions* (3rd ed.). Chicago, IL: University of Chicago Press. (Original work published 1962)

Latour, B. (1999). *Pandora's hope: Essays on the reality of science studies.* Cambridge, MA: Harvard University Press.

Latour, B., & Woolgar, S. (1986). *Laboratory life: The construction of scientific facts.* Princeton, NJ: Princeton University Press.

Lenoir, T. (1997). *Instituting science: The cultural production of scientific disciplines.* Stanford, CA: Stanford University Press.

Longino, H. E. (2002). *The fate of knowledge.* Princeton, NJ: Princeton University Press.

Lum, C. (2002). *Scientific thinking in speech and language therapy.* Mahwah, NJ: Lawrence Erlbaum.

Marrs, J., & Lowry, L. W. (2006). Nursing theory and practice: Connecting the dots. *Nursing Science Quarterly, 19*(2), 116–119.

Meleis, A. I., & Im, E. (1999). Transcending marginalization in knowledge development. *Nursing Inquiry, 6*(1), 94–102.

Montgomery, K. (2006). *How doctors think: Clinical judgment and the practice of medicine.* New York, NY: Oxford University Press.

Neill, J. (2005). Recognizing patterns in the lives of women with multiple sclerosis. In C. Picard & D. Jones (Eds.), *Giving voice to what we know* (pp. 153–168). Boston, MA: Jones & Bartlett.

Nelson, S., & Gordon, S. (Eds.). (2006). *The complexities of care: Nursing reconsidered.* Ithaca, NY: Cornell University Press.

Pickering, A. (1995). *The mangle of practice: Time, agency and science.* Chicago, IL: University of Chicago Press.

Purkis, M. E., & Bjornsdottir, K. (2006). Intelligent nursing: Accounting for knowledge as action *in* practice. *Nursing Philosophy, 7*, 247–256.

Rawnsley, M. M. (2000). Response to Leddy's "toward a complementary perspective on worldviews." *Nursing Science Quarterly, 13*, 230–233.

Reed, P. G. (1995). A treatise on nursing knowledge development for the 21st century: Beyond postmodernism. *Advances in Nursing Science, 17*(3), 70–84.

Reed, P. G. (2001, October). *An emancipatory model for knowledge development in nursing.* Paper presented at the Knowledge Impact Conference, Boston College School of Nursing, Boston, MA.

Reed, P. G. (2006). Commentary on neomodernism and evidence-based nursing: Implications for the production of nursing knowledge. *Nursing Outlook, 54*(1), 36–38.

Reed, P. G. (2011). The spiral path of nursing knowledge. In P. G. Reed & N. B. C. Shearer (Eds.), *Nursing knowledge and theory innovation advancing the science of practice* (pp. 1–35). New York, NY: Springer Publishing.

Reed, P. G. (2016). Epistemic authority in nursing practice vs. doctors' orders. *Nursing Science Quarterly, 29*(3), 241–246.

Reed, P. G., & Lawrence, L. A. (2008). A paradigm for the production of practice-based knowledge. *Journal of Nursing Management, 16*, 422–432.

Roberts, A. R., & Yeager, K. (2004). Systematic review of evidenced-based studies and practice-based research: How to search for, develop, and use them. In A. R. Roberts & K. Yeager (Eds.), *Evidence-based practice manual* (pp. 3–14). New York, NY: Oxford University Press.

Salas, A. S. (2005). Toward a North–South dialogue: Revisiting nursing theory (from the South). *Advances in Nursing Science, 28*(1), 17–24.

Seigfried, C. H. (1996). *Pragmatism and feminism: Reweaving the social fabric.* Chicago, IL: University of Chicago Press.

Serres, M. (1995). *Conversations on science, culture, and time: Michel Serres with Bruno Latour* (R. Lapidus, Trans.). Ann Arbor: University of Michigan Press.

Sturman, S. (2006). On black-boxing gender: Some social questions for Bruno Latour. *Social Epistemology, 20,* 181–184.

Thatchenkery, T., & Chowdhry, D. (2007). *Appreciative inquiry and knowledge management: A social constructionist perspective.* Northampton, MA: Edward Elgar.

Urban, A. (2013). Taken for granted: Normalizing nurses' work in hospitals. *Nursing Inquiry, 21*(1), 69–78.

U.S. Department of Health and Human Services and Health Resources and Services Administration. (2010). *The registered nurse population: Findings from the 2008 national sample survey of registered nurses.* Retrieved from https://datawarehouse.hrsa.gov/DataDownload/NSSRN/GeneralPUF08/rnsurveyfinal.pdf

14

Interlude V: *Steps in Reformulating a Nursing Practice Concept: Empowerment as an Example*[1]

Nelma B. Crawford Shearer and Pamela G. Reed

Concepts are critical elements in building knowledge. This chapter is intended to help you find a concept that you might be interested in exploring further through your studies or graduate research. Sometimes a concept of interest may be used or defined in a way that is not quite right by your judgment, beliefs, and experiences. Rather than abandon a potentially rich concept, you may reformulate (modify) the concept to fit your perspectives. This reformulation involves not only a sound literature review, but also reflecting on two important dimensions in your professional life: your nursing experiences and your philosophic views (worldviews) about human health and nursing practice.

There are many "not quite right" concepts in the literature that, with some reformulation according to your nursing perspective, may open a pathway to a new theory for nursing practice. The concept of empowerment presented in this chapter was a gateway to a theory about promoting the purposeful participation of homebound older women in their health and health care decisions. We invite you to read this

1. Adapted by permission of Sage Publications, Inc. from Shearer, N. B. C., & Reed, P. G. (2004). Empowerment: Reformulation of a non-Rogerian concept. *Nursing Science Quarterly, 17*(3), 253–259.

chapter as an example of concept reformulation and then experiment with your own ideas about potential concepts related to practice for inquiry.

Reformulation of the concept of empowerment emerged from my experiences in practice, a Rogerian worldview, and ideas gleaned through concept analysis and clarification conducted in graduate course work. The following excerpt is an example of a practice experience that inspired the idea of reformulating the concept of empowerment so as to emphasize a participative, not paternalistic, approach to helping individuals recognize and engage in changing their health patterns.

> I listened to the audio-tapes recorded for my research project while the nurses participating in the telephone intervention study talked and listened to the participants. Listening to the tapes has been an education in itself. While reviewing the tapes, it became apparent that one of the nurses making the telephone calls does not listen to the participant although I am sure she would strongly disagree with me. She is bent on getting the study participant to exercise and drink water. One participant in particular refers to listening to her body and states, "I know when something is wrong." The nurse responds by telling her she should instead talk with her doctor.
>
> (Notes Recorded by a Rogerian Research Nurse, March 18, 2002)

The lack of knowledge and misuse of power in health care by the nurse may not only reduce the individual's power to participate in his or her own health process but also diminish the nurse's own power as a facilitator of health care. I identified empowerment as a theoretical concept of potential relevance to facilitating a person's participation in his or her own health care. But I wanted to conceptualize it from within my philosophical perspective of nursing practice. This required some reformulation of traditional use of the concept.

PHILOSOPHICAL RATIONALE FOR REFORMULATING

From a philosophy of science perspective, modifying (or reformulating) existing concepts, ideas, or theories is an accepted practice in science. Philosophers support this as an approach to knowledge development. Nurse theoretician Whall (1980), drawing from philosopher of science Kaplan's (1964) ideas on the autonomy of inquiry, instructed scholars that concepts and theories are not owned by any one discipline and may be reformulated according to their own disciplinary perspectives and purposes.

From a moral perspective, it may be wise to reformulate rather than *ignore* or continue using concepts and theories that are incongruent with a disciplinary perspective. As nurses, we believed in the benefits of a nursing perspective in health care and thought that the attitude conveyed by the nurse in the notes previously conflicted with good nursing care. In this case, for example, reformulating the concept of empowerment was an opportunity to clarify and suggest new thinking about a fairly common approach to positively influence nurses' everyday interactions with patients.

After considering rationale for reformulating empowerment and determining it was an important phase in developing a theory of health empowerment (Shearer, 2007), several steps were followed. We describe each step briefly and then elaborate on our work as an example of the step. The general focus of each of these steps can be applied to modifying other concepts.

STEPS IN REFORMULATING
A CONCEPT

Reformulation involves a series of steps, beginning with the existing concept and concluding with the reformulated concept. It begins with a clarification about the author's philosophic views about nursing and human health, as they influence what ideas are used to modify the concept. Reformulation also includes a review of basic definitions of the concept, historical perspectives, and paradigmatic views from various disciplines that influence current thought on empowerment. A review of the research literature and a concept analysis may also be conducted early on in the reformulation. Next, the assumptions and principles of relevant nursing and nonnursing theories are considered. It is also an important step to critically address the nursing practice paradigms that may influence translation of the concept into action.

STEP 1. CLARIFY YOUR PERSPECTIVE OF NURSING

Clarifying our theoretical perspective was useful in synthesizing a coherent and philosophically relevant reformulation of empowerment out of the wide variety of theories (nursing and nonnursing) about the concept. The reformulation was based on Rogerian nursing principles (Rogers, 1980, 1990, 1992) and the shift from positivist philosophy to philosophic views that supported a participative approach of helping individuals recognize and engage in changing their health patterns.

Rogers (1980, 1990, 1992) defined nursing's focus as the study of human beings in mutual process with the environment. Rogers proposed three principles of homeodynamics, which outline her assumptions about the nature of the human–environment process as well as guide nursing practice. The principle of helicy describes the nature of human change as continuous, innovative, unpredictable, and reflective of the diversity of human and environment patterns. The principle of integrality proposes how this change occurs, that is, through a continuous mutual process of human and environmental systems. The idea is that human beings and environment evolve in action together rather than as separate entities in reaction against each other. The principle of resonancy emphasizes the existence of patterns rather than parts that characterize human beings and their environment. Knowledge about these patterns is acquired through research and careful assessment and can then be used to facilitate health.

STEP 2. EXAMINE AND EVALUATE EXISTING DEFINITIONS AND DESCRIPTIONS OF THE CONCEPT

Empowerment is a ubiquitous concept not only in the health care literature but also across many social disciplines. In general, it connotes active participation in one's own health care. Furthermore, moral views and behaviors, personal integrity, and a sense of personal and social responsibility have been found to be qualities of empowerment (Kuokkanen, Leino-Kilpi, & Katajisto, 2002). Empowerment is generally associated with increased self-esteem and self-worth, inner confidence and strength, and well-being (e.g., Dowling, Murphy, Cooney, & Casey, 2011; Gibson, 1991; Kieffer, 1984; Nyatanga & Dann, 2002).

Barrett, Caroselli, Smith, and Smith (1997) pointed out that the term's literal definition, to *put power into* an individual, reflects a mechanistic view of human beings in terms of the person passively receiving something from another. The definition also suggests an authoritative view of nursing, with the nurse as the primary one with the power and authority. Both of these views were evaluated as being incongruent with a nursing perspective, particularly given Rogers's (1980, 1990, 1992) descriptions of human beings and nursing practice.

STEP 3. REVIEW THE HISTORY OF THE CONCEPT

According to Minkler and Wallerstein (1997), the word *empowerment* first appeared in the literature during the 1950s, a time of social action organization in which the emphasis was on addressing power imbalances. Empowerment rooted in social action became more influential throughout the 1960s and 1970s within the contexts of civil rights, the women's movement, gay rights, the disability rights movement, and other community-based action. During the 1980s, in the psychology literature, empowerment was viewed as a participatory process through which individuals take control over their lives and environment (Rappaport, 1984). It was not until the 1990s, when health care providers' and consumers' focus turned to health promotion that the concept appeared on a regular basis in the nursing and health education literature.

In the context of health education, empowerment has been viewed as a process and an outcome; as a process, empowerment involves relationships and the transfer of the power base from one group to another, with the outcome of "liberation, emancipation, energy and sharing power" (Leyshon, 2002, p. 467). In the context of nursing, empowerment has been understood from various broad perspectives; "adoption of empowerment largely rested on abstract theoretical concepts which were adopted with basic understanding of their meaning" (Chambers & Thompson, 2009, p. 132).

STEP 4. REVIEW CURRENT PERSPECTIVES, ASSUMPTIONS, AND THEORIES RELATED TO THE CONCEPT

Given nursing's basic assumptions about the importance of human potential and development, connectedness, and the social context in health and well-being, both the social and developmental paradigms offer ideas that are useful in reformulating the concept of empowerment.

Social Paradigms

As a social process, empowerment is linked with external social forces that act on the individual and affect one's sense of control and feelings of power. For example, social support as an external feedback mechanism has been studied as a process that can provide needed reinforcement, resources, assistance, and motivation (Ellis-Stoll & Popkess-Vawter, 1998) and enable the individual (Hawks, 1992). Other external social forces have been studied from the perspective of emancipation from oppression. Several authors have suggested that promoting empowerment could be accomplished through addressing political (Gutierrez, 1995; Labonte, 1994), environmental (Ryles, 1999), and social constraints (Fulton, 1997). Two theories addressing these constraints are critical social theory and feminist theory, which offer perspectives about power applicable in nursing.

Critical social theory evolved from Marxism during the postmodern era and from the revolutionary thinking of Paulo Freire (1968/1981) in Brazil. Freire's basic assumption is that human being's "ontological vocation is to be a Subject who acts upon and transforms one's world" (Richard Shaull, as cited in Freire, 1968/1981, p. 12). The goals of critical social theory are to make people aware of the social constraints under which they may be consciously or unconsciously living, free people's thinking, and establish unconstrained communication.

Feminist thought of the 1960s extended the suffragists' cause of the late 19th through early 20th century to address the educational, occupational, professional, and role-related constraints experienced by women. Although diverse views on feminism exist, a unifying theme is the elimination of patriarchal social constraints and the oppression of women (Kirkley, 2000). Feminist theory acknowledges basic human potential in all human beings and incorporates interactions and life experiences that contribute to human transformation; this transformation of oppressive situations facilitates empowerment (Kane & Thomas, 2000). Empowerment from a feminist perspective draws from the ideology of equality by emphasizing the choices and freedom of women (Caroselli, 1995).

In addition, *postmodern feminism* has introduced a multicultural and global focus in which differences in race, class, national origin, and gender are regarded as relevant in the discourse on constraints on women's freedom and well-being (Tong, 2001). Postcolonial feminist theory has shifted away from the earlier emphasis on achieving a unified notion of women toward developing an appreciation of differences while holding a collective goal of equal opportunity. There is less of a stance of victimization and a more creative, proactive approach to one's social environment that develops the human potential of all (Ramphele, 1997).

Developmental Paradigm

Empowerment may also be understood in reference to the life-span developmental perspective that emerged in the late 1970s (Lerner, 1997). Life-span development is an orientation to the study of human beings as continuously innovative, embedded in a dynamic environment, and possessing inherent potential. The life-span developmental perspective emphasizes both *systematic* patterns of change, such as biologically based influences, and *nonnormative* patterns of change across the life span, such as life events that cannot be predicted by time and do not occur for everyone. Development is no longer viewed as a linear process as it was until the late 20th century. Rather, developmental change is now understood to derive unpredictably from mutual influences between person and environmental contexts. Person–environment processes, including those involving human relationships, are central to developmental progress and well-being.

Treatment approaches from a life-span view focus on maximizing strengths and minimizing weaknesses (Baltes, Lindenberger, & Staudinger, 1998) rather than on predetermined interventions designed to change behaviors. The individual is regarded as possessing a repertoire of developmentally based abilities that can be educed through the nurse–person relationship to address health care needs. From this perspective, the individual is a resource and active partner in health care. Nursing care is directed less toward changing the person and more toward optimizing human potential.

Related Nursing Theories

Several theoretical frameworks support the Rogerian postulate that people desire to participate knowingly in change and in their patterning. This idea has a central place in Barrett et al.'s (1997) power enhancement, Newman's (1997) expanding consciousness, and Reed's (1997) participatory nursing process. Synthesis of ideas from these frameworks supports a reformulation of the concept of empowerment.

BARRETT. Barrett's (1990, 2010) theory of *power as knowing participation in change* is similar to, but still qualitatively different from, typical views of empowerment. Barrett's underlying assumption about participation in ongoing change is a unique perspective. Basic to Barrett's (1990, 1994, 2010) theory of power is the assumption of ongoing change and the individual's awareness of and belief in one's ability to fully participate in the changes involved in health and health care. The partnership with the nurse facilitates the individual's participation in health care. During the health-seeking event, the participatory relationship evolves. The nurse uses various methods that enhance the person's knowing participation in change. One such approach centers on finding out what is happening with the individual, directing attention away from the nurse as the initiator of nursing care and toward a participatory relationship in which both facilitate the change process. The nursing goal is "power enhancement through changing the environment" (Barrett et al., 1997, p. 34).

NEWMAN. Newman's (1997) theory of health as expanding consciousness proposes a mutual process by which the nurse facilitates individuals' insights and meaning of their own health patterns. The nurse does not attempt to control the interaction and change the person. Instead, the nurse facilitates pattern recognition and health choices (Newman, 1990). This process of pattern recognition expands the individual's developing insight and facilitates potential action.

REED. Reed (1997) described nursing as a "participatory process that transcends the boundary between patient and nurse" (p. 77). She defined nursing as an inherent process of well-being that functions within and among human systems. Reed explained that nursing, in its most basic meaning, is not an external process of 19th-century invention; rather, it is a resource that has existed among human beings ever since the beginning of human history. Empowerment is an expression and indicator of this inherent nursing process. From this participatory perspective, empowerment is inherent in the nurse–person system rather than located in either the nurse or the individual alone. The process promotes well-being through the resources inherent in this relational system.

STEP 5. REVIEW USES OF THE CONCEPT FROM THE PERSPECTIVES OF NURSING PRACTICE PARADIGMS

Parse (1987, 1992) identified two nursing paradigms, *totality* and *simultaneity*, that can guide thinking about nursing practice concepts. A Rogerian view of empowerment is congruent with the simultaneity paradigm of nursing practice. (More recently, Parse [2015] has described her "humanbecoming paradigm," which is consistent with the simultaneity view.)

Totality

According to the totality paradigm, humans are biopsychosocial–spiritual beings interacting with and in response to the internal and external environment (Parse, 1992). Human change is considered predictable, controllable, and occurring primarily in response to environmental stimuli. Health is viewed as achieving equilibrium in physical, mental, social, and spiritual dimensions. Within this paradigm, the nurse knows what is best for the individual and uses the nurse–person relationship to influence change in the desired direction. Empowerment is accomplished through the efforts of the nurse as data collector, assessor of the disease state, care planner, and change agent. The nurse as the authority shares knowledge to empower the individual to make informed choices that are appropriate and in compliance with the care plan.

Simultaneity

Within the simultaneity paradigm (Parse, 1992), human beings are recognized through pattern rather than through parts that can be independently manipulated, changed, and studied. Change is creative and innovative and occurs as part of the person–environment process. Health involves the individual's purposeful participation in developing self-awareness and choosing health patterns. People exercise their power by participating in their health care and health care decisions. The nurse's approach is to inspire, not dictate this process, and to be facilitative, not authoritative.

Uses of the Concept

It is not uncommon for health care providers to think that they can empower individuals and in so doing expect that they will comply with the health plan (e.g., Hawks, 1992; Holmes & Saleebey, 1993). Empowerment is often implicitly, if not explicitly, linked to the concept of compliance in practice. The concept neither appeals to the informed consumer nor reflects contemporary nursing philosophy of science. Clinical practice and anecdotal experiences consistently indicate that individuals do not always follow through with the nurse's prescribed plan of care (Hess, 1996). The nurse, thinking that the person has been amply empowered, may be puzzled as to why the person does not *comply* with the health care plan.

The confounding of empowerment and compliance is insidious and prevails even in literature appearing to advance understandings of empowerment beyond authoritarian assumptions, for example, "non-compliance demonstrated the patient's need to exercise their empowerment" (Nyatanga & Dann, 2002, p. 238), as though noncompliance really exists in patients and is linked to empowerment. The authors go on to explain that the nursing discipline should cease using the term *patients*, come around to the true philosophy of empowerment, and relinquish the discipline's authoritarian approach. However, the problem is not so much the lack of the correct understanding of empowerment as it is the nurse's practice paradigm (perspective) that influences applications of empowerment.

EMPOWERMENT REFORMULATED

Rogers did not specifically address empowerment in publications on her science of unitary human beings. Nonetheless, her theoretical views were helpful in synthesizing ideas from social and developmental theories. From Rogers (1992), it is understood that there is an emphasis on participating knowingly in the process of change rather than on submission and lack of power, control, or choice. Attention to external agents of power is inconsistent with these assumptions. The nurse is not one who empowers but rather one who facilitates empowerment in human beings, with actions deriving from an understanding of the person's relational nature, relevant social context, and developmental potential.

This new view of empowerment is based on four assumptions derived from Rogerian theory and related theories: (a) Empowerment is neither a resource that is external to the person nor bestowed by others; power is inherent and ongoing (Labonte, 1989); (b) Empowerment is a relational process, expressive of the mutuality of person and environment; (c) Empowerment is an ongoing process of change that is continuously innovative; and (d) Empowerment is expressive of a human health pattern of well-being and can be assessed and enhanced through nursing knowledge, including practice and science-based inquiry.

Empowerment as reformulated, then, is defined as *a health patterning of well-being in which the individual optimizes the ability to transform self through the relational process of nursing*. It may involve identifying and transcending sources of oppression that constrain human potential and limit self-understanding of personal resources. The Rogerian ideas of Barrett et al.'s (1997) power enhancement, Newman's (1997) expanding consciousness, and Reed's (1997) participatory process of well-being together provide for a reformulated view of empowerment—one that extends the possibilities of change for all participants (Cowling, 2001) as a dynamic human health process. Empowerment can then be understood as a complex and participatory process of changing oneself and one's environment, recognizing patterns, and engaging inner resources for well-being. It is a process greater than any one theory can represent. It is a process that is central to a unitary perspective of human beings (Cowling, 2001).

A CASE STUDY

The following story illustrates the experience of empowerment and offers an example of the mutual process of power that is inherent in the nurse–person system. Rachel, a community health nurse, focuses on patterning the environment with Patricia to promote Patricia's sense of power to participate in health care and health care decisions. In their interactions, Rachel focuses on Patricia's strengths, is supportive, and provides empowering education that promotes Patricia's health.

Several years ago, Rachel met Patricia during a home visit. Patricia was in her late 70s and was diagnosed with chronic obstructive pulmonary disease (COPD), osteoporosis, and heart failure. She was on many medications, including nebulizer treatments, inhalers, continuous oxygen, and pills. Patricia had been in the hospital frequently for COPD exacerbations. She told Rachel that she did not like going to the hospital: "They didn't do much for me other than increasing my breathing treatments and giving me IV steroids," and "I can do that at home."

Patricia lived with her son, daughter-in-law, and their two children. She had an upstairs bedroom and stayed there except for meals, which she would take down in the kitchen if her breathing would allow it. She said the family did not provide her with much support, and often she would go for days without anyone coming in to say "hi." Patricia was lonely. She filled her time with crafts including crocheting and making items with beads, plus she liked to read and watch video movies. She told Rachel she did not know where a couple of her children were and she had a daughter in prison for armed robbery. She communicated with this daughter through letters and they provided each other with support.

When they first met, Patricia was a little skeptical of Rachel's ability. She told Rachel later that she did not know what a nurse would be able to do for her and that she had been used to taking care of herself and her own health. They discussed Patricia's health, and Rachel provided her with information on ways that she could take care of herself so she would not have frequent exacerbations and end up in the hospital. They talked about daily weighing and she got permission from the physician to take extra Lasix if her weight increased. Patricia and Rachel talked about Patricia's frequent breathing crises and the importance of catching things early, listening to her body, and being in tune with her breathing pattern. Increasingly, Patricia became more *in tune* with her body and more aware of when she needed to call the physician for an antibiotic or an increase in prednisone to prevent further complications.

Patricia developed moon face and was also having neck pain from the damage that had been caused by taking prednisone. She wanted to stop taking it, but whenever she asked the physician he said, "No." Patricia and Rachel talked about it, and Rachel supported her in her efforts. They talked about the risks (and the benefits) of being off prednisone, and Patricia made her decision. She weaned herself off very gradually and was successful in staying off except when she would get a bad cold or infection.

Patricia began to feel so good that she began to verbalize that perhaps she could get out of her children's hair and get her own place. Patricia and Rachel talked about her options, including the possibility of moving into a group home or an assisted living arrangement. Unfortunately, due to Patricia's limited income, she was unable to move from her children's home, but she decided that she could get out of the house during the day to participate in group activities. Rachel and Patricia visited two senior centers and determined together which one had programs that fit Patricia's interests.

Rachel no longer has Patricia as a client. Patricia moved out of state and lives with her daughter. Rachel shared that she learned a great deal from Patricia, especially about the importance of a person actively participating in the ongoing changes in her health and the ever-present potential for well-being.

> Patricia told me she appreciated that I encouraged her to participate in the decisions regarding her own life and health. But really what happened was that Patricia became aware of her ability to actively participate in making health decisions. She just needed to be educated on a better way of handling things and then needed the support to do it. She taught me what it is like to live with chronic illness and yet look forward to every day.

Thus, Patricia was empowered by this participatory mutual process in which the nurse nurtured Patricia's ability to recognize her pattern of well-being and her natural resources for healing self. In addition, Rachel was empowered by facilitating the mutual process of innovative change for Patricia.

CONCLUSIONS

Rogerian science was used to synthesize a new view of empowerment out of social and developmental perspectives. The reformulation is consistent with nursing assumptions about patterns of human health and change. It is also congruent with the simultaneity paradigm of nursing practice. Reformulation of the concept involved a shift in focus from empowerment *for* individuals to the relational process of empowerment within and among human systems, nurse and person alike.

This shift in thinking that occurred at a concept level has yet to be fully realized in nursing practice. The proposed view alters the traditional paternalistic focus in health care systems that minimizes the individual's identity, choice, and participation in health, and in so doing minimizes the role of nursing overall.

Empowerment represents a dynamic human health process, one of many that nursing seeks to understand for the betterment of society. By enacting a worldview that acknowledges empowerment as a nursing process inherent in and among human beings, nurses relinquish an authoritarian nursing process external to the person. Nurses and individuals may work together more equally and effectively to promote health and well-being, thereby moving nursing from the practice to the praxis of empowerment.

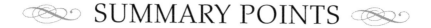

SUMMARY POINTS

1. Concept reformulation aids in clarifying an existing concept into one that is congruent with a nursing perspective.

2. Concept reformulation is often an initial activity in theory development, especially with concepts borrowed from other disciplines or contexts different from nursing practice.

3. Reformulation involves specific steps, including consideration of the nurse's own philosophical perspective.

4. The nursing discipline has distinct philosophical perspectives that can guide concept reformulation.

 # QUESTIONS FOR REFLECTION

1. What concept interests you as related to your nursing practice? Think about how you might decide on a concept related to practice.

2. How would you define your concept according to your knowledge and views about human health and nursing practice?

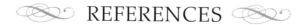 # REFERENCES

Baltes, P. B., Lindenberger, U., & Staudinger, U. M. (1998). Life-span theory in developmental psychology. In R. Lerner (Ed.), *Theoretical models of human development* (pp. 1029–1143). New York, NY: Wiley.

Barrett, E. A. M. (1990). Health patterning with clients in a private practice environment. In E. A. M. Barrett (Ed.), *Visions of Rogers' science-based nursing* (pp. 105–115). New York, NY: National League for Nursing.

Barrett, E. A. M. (1994). Rogerian scientists, artists, revolutionaries. In M. Madrid & E. A. M. Barrett (Eds.), *Rogers' scientific art of nursing practice* (pp. 61–87). New York, NY: National League for Nursing.

Barrett, E. A. M. (2010). Power as knowing participation in change: What's new and what's next. *Nursing Science Quarterly, 23,* 47–54.

Barrett, E. A. M., Caroselli, C., Smith, A. S., & Smith, D. W. (1997). Power as knowing participation in change: Theoretical, practice, and methodological issues, insights, and ideas. In M. Madrid (Ed.), *Patterns of Rogerian knowing* (pp. 31–46). New York, NY: National League for Nursing.

Caroselli, C. (1995). Power and feminism: A nursing science perspective. *Nursing Science Quarterly, 8,* 115–119.

Chambers, D., & Thompson, S. (2009). Empowerment and its application in health promotion in acute care settings: Nurses' perceptions. *Journal of Advanced Nursing, 65,* 130–138.

Cowling, W. R. (2001). Unitary appreciative inquiry. *Advances in Nursing Science, 23*(4), 32–48.

Dowling, M., Murphy, K., Cooney, A., & Casey, D. (2011). A concept analysis of empowerment in chronic illness from the nurse and the client living with chronic obstructive pulmonary disease. *Journal of Nursing and Healthcare of Chronic Illness, 3,* 476–487.

Ellis-Stoll, C., & Popkess-Vawter, S. (1998). A concept analysis on the process of empowerment. *Advances in Nursing Science, 21*(2), 62–68.

Freire, P. (1981). *Pedagogy of the oppressed* (M. B. Ramos, Trans.). New York, NY: Continuum. (Original work published 1968)

Fulton, Y. (1997). Nurses' views on empowerment: A critical social theory perspective. *Journal of Advanced Nursing, 26,* 529–536.

Gibson, C. H. (1991). A concept analysis of empowerment. *Journal of Advanced Nursing, 16,* 354–361.

Gutierrez, L. (1995). Understanding the empowerment process: Does consciousness make a difference? *Social Work Research, 19,* 229–237.

Hawks, J. (1992). Empowerment in nursing education: Concept analysis and application to philosophy, learning and instruction. *Journal of Advanced Nursing, 17,* 609–618.

Hess, J. (1996). The ethics of compliance: A dialectic. *Advances in Nursing Science, 19*(1), 18–27.

Holmes, G., & Saleebey, D. (1993). Empowerment, the medical model, and the politics of clienthood. *Journal of Progressive Human Services, 4*(1), 61–78.

Kane, D., & Thomas, B. (2000). Nursing and the "F" word. *Nursing Forum, 35*(2), 17–24.

Kaplan, A. (1964). *The conduct of inquiry.* New York, NY: Thomas Y. Crowell.

Kieffer, C. (1984). Citizen empowerment: A developmental perspective. *Prevention in Human Services, 3,* 9–36.

Kirkley, D. (2000). Is motherhood good for women? A feminist exploration. *Journal of Obstetrics, Gynecologic and Neonatal Nursing, 29,* 459–464.

Kuokkanen, L., Leino-Kilpi, H., & Katajisto, J. (2002). Do nurses feel empowered? Nurses' assessment of their own qualities and performance with regard to nurse empowerment. *Journal of Professional Nursing, 18,* 328–335.

Labonte, R. (1989). Community and professional empowerment. *Canadian Nurse, 85*(3), 22–28.

Labonte, R. (1994). Health promotion and empowerment: Reflections on professional practice. *Health Education Quarterly, 21,* 253–268.

Lerner, R. (1997). *Concepts and theories of human development* (2nd ed.). Mahwah, NJ: Lawrence Erlbaum.

Leyshon, S. (2002). Empowering practitioners: An unrealistic expectation of nurse education? *Journal of Advanced Nursing, 40,* 466–474.

Minkler, M., & Wallerstein, N. (1997). Improving health through community organization and community building. In K. Glanz, F. Lewis, & B. Rimer (Eds.), *Health behavior and health education: Theory, research, and practice* (2nd ed., pp. 241–269). San Francisco, CA: Jossey-Bass.

Newman, M. (1990). Shifting to higher consciousness. In M. Parker (Ed.), *Nursing theories in practice* (pp. 129–139). New York, NY: National League for Nursing.

Newman, M. (1997). Evolution of the theory of health as expanding consciousness. *Nursing Science Quarterly, 10,* 22–25.

Nyatanga, L., & Dann, K. L. (2002). Empowerment in nursing: The role of philosophical and psychological factors. *Nursing Philosophy, 3,* 234–239.

Parse, R. R. (1987). Paradigms and theories. In R. R. Parse (Ed.), *Nursing science: Major paradigms, theories, and critiques* (pp. 1–11). Philadelphia, PA: Saunders.

Parse, R. R. (1992). Human becoming: Parse's theory of nursing. *Nursing Science Quarterly, 5,* 35–42.

Parse, R. R. (2015). Rosemarie Rizzo Parse's human becoming paradigm. In M. C. Cmith & M. E. Parker (Eds.), *Nursing theories & nursing practice* (4th ed., pp. 263–277). Philadelphia, PA: F. A. Davis.

Ramphele, M. (1997). Whither feminism? In J. Scott, C. Kaplan, & D. Keates (Eds.), *Transitions, environments, translations* (pp. 334–338). New York, NY: Routledge.

Rappaport, J. (1984). Studies in empowerment: Introduction to the issue. *Prevention in Human Services, 3*(2/3), 1–7.

Reed, P. G. (1997). Nursing: The ontology of the discipline. *Nursing Science Quarterly, 10,* 76–79.

Rogers, M. E. (1980). A science of unitary man. In J. P. Riehl & C. Roy (Eds.), *Conceptual models for nursing practice* (2nd ed., pp. 329–337). New York, NY: Appleton-Century-Crofts.

Rogers, M. E. (1990). Nursing: Science of unitary, irreducible, human beings: Update 1990. In E. A. M. Barrett (Ed.), *Visions of Rogers' science-based nursing* (pp. 5–11). New York, NY: National League for Nursing.

Rogers, M. E. (1992). Nursing science and space age. *Nursing Science Quarterly, 5,* 27–34.

Ryles, S. (1999). A concept analysis of empowerment: Its relationship to mental health nursing. *Journal of Advanced Nursing, 29,* 600–607.

Shearer, N. B. C. (2007). Toward a nursing theory of health empowerment in home-bound older women. *Journal of Gerontological Nursing, 33*(12), 38–45.

Shearer, N. B. C., & Reed, P. G. (2004). Empowerment: Reformulation of a non-Rogerian concept. *Nursing Science Quarterly, 17*(3), 253–259.

Tong, R. (2001). A millennial feminist vision. In J. P. Sterba (Ed.), *Controversies in feminism* (pp. 173–195). Lanham, MD: Rowman & Littlefield.

Whall, A. (1980). Congruence between existing theories of family functioning and nursing theories. *Advances in Nursing Science, 3*(1), 59–67.

The Practice Turn and Nursing Theory Innovation[1]

Pamela G. Reed

This chapter brings the book to an end by revisiting an idea that initiated this book, that is, the idea that nursing knowledge development is integral with nursing practice, wherever it occurs as a process of facilitating human health and well-being. Nursing practice typically has been viewed as a *context for applying* knowledge or theory but not as a *process of developing* knowledge and theory. With the shift in the educational philosophy toward increasing the numbers of graduate-level nurses, nursing has an opportunity to extend knowledge-production resources into nursing practice. For this to happen, though, there needs to be an accompanying shift in our philosophy of knowledge development in nursing.

The *turn* in this chapter refers to a change in focus—one that expands the traditional approach to linking theory and practice in *theory-guided practice* to include a focus on *practice-guided theory development*. With this philosophic perspective about knowledge (i.e., epistemology), nurses may engage in theory development that is more context relevant and *patient centered*. As you read, I invite you to reflect on these ideas in reference to your own nursing practice.

1. Adapted with permission of Sage Publications, Inc. from Reed P. G. (2006). The practice turn in nursing epistemology. *Nursing Science Quarterly, 19*(1), 36–38.

Nursing is a fascinating discipline. Nurses have both the honor and expertise to participate closely in human healing processes of individuals, families, and communities. Yet, because the practitioner's expertise in healing is not fully understood, some account for it by relying on concepts, like intuition, tacit knowing, and gut feelings, that render nursing knowledge more mystical than professional. Admittedly, there are elements of mystery in nurses' patterns of knowing, just as there is mystery that accompanies scientific knowledge in general (e.g., Adam, 2009; Raymo, 2006). However, contrary to philosophers of science Reichenbach and Popper, the *context of discovery* is not primarily mystical territory. I think it is both possible and beneficial to pursue fuller explanations of how nursing knowledge is produced in the context of practice. Furthermore, trends in practice regarding evidence-based nursing, an intensified interest in advanced practice degrees, and the rise of the doctor of nursing practice degree all necessitate inquiry into nursing's epistemological infrastructure. So in this chapter, I have proposed rationale and a model for thinking anew about theory innovation and knowledge production in nursing practice.

For too long, nurses and other practicing professionals have more or less accepted the idea of a theory–practice gap and viewed science as distinct from a discipline's art or practice. The researcher has been portrayed as the *producer* who hands down scientific knowledge to the clinician as the *applier* of knowledge, sometimes *supplier* of ideas or researchable problems, maybe even *tester* of knowledge, but rarely *producer* of knowledge and theory. This traditional model of nursing knowledge production may not only misrepresent and constrain the knowledge potential in nursing but also marginalize the practitioner and distance patients from the process of knowledge development. There is a need for philosophical inquiry into beliefs and values about the "truest" or best source of nursing knowledge. In addition, there is a need for empirical inquiry into whether and how nurses produce knowledge through their practice. The results are likely to extend the science of nursing practice well beyond descriptions of intuition or gut feelings and even beyond current descriptions of critical thinking and clinical reasoning.

Granted, knowledge from nursing and other sciences developed outside of nursing practice can be useful for application, perhaps with needed translation or reformulation. However, to the extent that nurses strive to facilitate patients' resources and participation in care and healing processes, it seems logical to include if not emphasize—over the researcher-centered model—a nurse–patient practice-centered model in developing scientific knowledge. For example, knowledge generated through practice can more effectively address the thorny epistemological question of "Who can speak for others?" (Alcoff, 1995) by enabling the nurse to speak not *for* the patient but *with* the patient.

Precursors to this *practice turn*—as originally labeled by Rouse (2002) and others (e.g., Schatzki, Cetina, & von Savigny, 2001)—in epistemology were evident in nursing more than a half-century ago. In addition, during the last decade, scholars within and outside of nursing increasingly acknowledged the role of human practices in knowledge production and critiqued orthodox epistemology with its one path to scientific knowledge.

NURSING

Mining our nursing history for ideas about nursing knowledge in the conceptual models and theorists' publications turned up several statements where scholars had specifically described practitioners as producers of theory and knowledge. More than 50 years ago, Peplau (1952, 1992) presented her *cycle of inquiry* whereby the practitioner transformed practice knowledge into nursing knowledge. Peplau (1952, 1992) explained that the practicing nurse peels out theoretical explanations and formulates hypotheses, which are then validated and tested in the context of the nurse–patient relationship (Reed, 1996). Ellis (1969) conceptualized the *practitioner as theorist* and plainly stated that the practitioner was "not simply a user of given theory but a developer, tester, and expander of theory" (p. 1438).

Paterson and Zderad (1976) outlined five phases in nursology, the phenomenological study of nursing practice. Researcher and practitioner roles were integrated and nurse–patient interactions produced theoretical *conceptions* derived from the local situation that held meaning across multiple situations. Roy and Obloy (1978) described the practitioner as building knowledge through practice and, in fact, defined this as the process of nursing science. Diers's (1995) seminal work on clinical scholarship paved a way for practitioners to raise their clinical observations and stories to the "level of theory" (p. 27). The next century brought an increasing number of nursing publications focused on nursing praxis as the *inseparability of theory/practice* (e.g., Connor, 2004; Doane & Varcoe, 2005; Rolfe, 1996, 2000).

SCIENCE STUDIES

Outside of nursing, sociology and culture scholars from the field of science studies (see Hess, 1997, for an overview) and the writings by historians and philosophers of science indirectly provided vigorous support for promoting nursing practice as integral to nursing knowledge and theory production. For example, Gibbons et al. (1994) proposed the now popular Mode 2 form of knowledge production that supplements traditional Mode 1 research approaches. Within the Mode 2 approach, knowledge evolves close to the *context of application* and, in fact, knowledge is legitimized by its use. Pickstone (2000) theorized that ways of knowing are linked to one's work and ways of making things. The practice-centered philosophy of Shusterman (1997) suggested that the embodied experiences of practicing and receiving nursing care, and then reflecting on these events, comprise a process that generates new knowledge. In addition, Baird's (2004) philosophic inquiry into technology established important links between the intelligent use of instruments in practice and scientific knowledge. So a nurse's interface with technology in patient care provides another opportunity for knowledge production in the context of practice.

In addition, historians have clarified that science itself is a practice and one that is much messier than what is portrayed in traditional descriptions of research. For example, Pickering (1995) described science as a *mangle* of social, technical, conceptual, political, and personal practices. *Is this not descriptive of our science of nursing practice?*

It is uncertain whether practicing nurses will embrace the practice turn in epistemology. Nevertheless, findings from Abbott's (1988) research into professions indicate that practitioners and the profession as a whole would benefit from theory-based knowledge production in practice. From his widely cited study of professions, Abbott concluded that *abstract thinking* was a dominant factor in determining whether professions had full jurisdiction over their practice. He identified nursing as an exemplar of a profession with limited jurisdiction, implying that nursing lacked sufficient activity of abstract thinking in practice. *Is this still so?* Or do nurses peel out concepts and theories from their interactions with patients to produce practice knowledge? A study by Larsen, Adamsen, Bjerregaard, and Madsen (2002) found that clinical nurses identified various sources of knowledge but denied using or producing theory in their practice. *Is this still the case?*

TOWARD A NEW MODEL OF THEORY INNOVATION AND KNOWLEDGE PRODUCTION

I suggest that knowledge production be conceptualized as integral with practice, patient centered, and theory based, and that practicing nurses be viewed as eminently capable of integrating theoretical thinking with data from patient interactions to develop knowledge and theories relevant to patient care. Theorizing in practice is a creative process that can be studied, taught, and facilitated. To theorize is to think abstractly and make links between the empirical and conceptual. Practitioners who function as theory-based knowledge producers can help bring about the discipline's realization of full jurisdiction over nursing practice.

This model does not exclude the role of traditional research in knowledge production. Partnerships between practitioners and researchers still hold. However, practice-based research methods need to be taught in practice-doctorate curricula more deliberately, more thoroughly, and with conviction in the practicing nurse as a producer of knowledge. Further, I propose that the nursing researcher who typically practices science without direct experience in nursing practice produces knowledge *of* nursing, employing systematic methods of scientific inquiry that emphasize the empirical patterns of knowing. The practitioner, however, practices science within the context of nursing care and produces knowledge *in* nursing by employing a wider array of patterns of knowing (aesthetic, ethical, technological, and including empirical) to generate nursing theories.

Three basic assumptions underlie this model of knowledge production and theory innovation. They are as follows:

1. Nursing practice is a process of facilitating human processes of health and well-being.

2. The nursing practice setting is not only a place of knowledge application, but also a context wherein nurse–patient encounters generate important data for building nursing knowledge.

3. Knowledge building involves abstract thought and generation or refinement of nursing theory, at some level of theory.

CONCLUSIONS

The characterizations of practitioner and researcher roles and other ideas that I have suggested in this chapter admittedly will benefit from more thought and dialogue, and from research! The model begs for explanations about whether and how practicing nurses engage in roles of both practitioners and researchers to produce theory-based knowledge. Part of the answer lies in examining existing descriptions and theories about the various forms of human reasoning. Part of the answer will come from systematic study of practitioners and other caregivers in their daily work. And part of the answer resides in the philosophy, goals, and values nurses have about their science and practice.

There is increasing evidence in the literature of a convergence of thought occurring simultaneously and independently across scholars—a phenomenon Lamb and Easton (1984) called *multiple discoveries*—about nursing practice and knowledge. In other words, multiple people are expressing similar ideas about the significance of practice in the production of nursing knowledge and theory. I hope more nurses will consider the untapped role of practice in nursing theory innovation and knowledge production, will question traditional views of science that may subordinate clinicians' expert knowing, and will turn scholarly attention toward exploring what it means to know and who are the legitimate knowers in nursing. May more nurses join the multiple discoveries unfolding to advance the state of knowledge and theory production in nursing practice and to advance the status of the discipline and its capacity to facilitate human health and well-being.

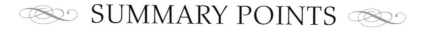

SUMMARY POINTS

1. The *practice turn* in nursing knowledge development—accompanied by a similar shift in philosophy of science—refers to an expansion of the traditional approach to linking theory and practice in *theory-guided practice* to include a focus on *practice-guided theory development.*

2. Nursing scholars across our discipline's history promoted practitioners as developers as well as users of nursing theory and scientific knowledge.

3. A major assumption underlying the proposed model of knowledge production and theory innovation is that knowledge production involves abstract thought and generation or refinement of nursing theory.

4. There is a convergence of thought called *multiple discoveries* whereby multiple people are simultaneously expressing similar ideas about the significance of practice in the production of nursing knowledge and theory innovation.

 # QUESTIONS FOR REFLECTION

1. What role should nursing practice have in nursing theory innovation and knowledge development?

2. What changes are needed to support nurses' knowledge-development activities in practice?

3. What changes need to occur in nursing education to facilitate development of practicing nurses as theory builders?

4. What new (and existing) research strategies and methods can be used to build knowledge and theory in practice?

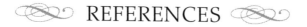 # REFERENCES

Abbott, A. (1988). *The system of professions.* Chicago, IL: University of Chicago Press.

Adam, F. (2009). *The constant fire: Beyond the science vs. religion debate.* Berkeley: University of California Press.

Alcoff, L. M. (1995). The problem of speaking for others. In J. Roof & R. Wiegman (Eds.), *Who can speak? Authority and critical identity* (pp. 97–119). Chicago: University of Illinois Press.

Baird, D. (2004). *Thing knowledge: A philosophy of scientific instruments*. Los Angeles: University of California Press.

Connor, M. J. (2004). The practical discourse in philosophy and nursing: An exploration of linkages and shifts in the evolution of praxis. *Nursing Philosophy, 5*, 54–66.

Diers, D. (1995). Clinical scholarship. *Journal of Professional Nursing, 11*(1), 24–30.

Doane, G. H., & Varcoe, C. (2005). Toward compassionate action: Pragmatism and the inseparability of theory/practice. *Advances in Nursing Science, 28*(1), 81–90.

Ellis, R. (1969). The practitioner as theorist. *American Journal of Nursing, 68*, 1434–1438.

Gibbons, M., Limoges, C., Nowotny, H., Schwartzman, S., Scott, P., & Trow, M. (1994). *The new production of knowledge: The dynamics of science and research in contemporary societies*. Thousand Oaks, CA: Sage.

Hess, D. J. (1997). *Science studies: An advanced introduction*. New York: New York University Press.

Lamb, D., & Easton, S. M. (1984). *Multiple discovery: The pattern of scientific progress*. Trowbridge, United Kingdom: Avebury.

Larsen, K., Adamsen, L., Bjerregaard, L., & Madsen, J. K. (2002). There is no gap "per se" between theory and practice: Research knowledge and clinical knowledge are developed in different contexts and follow their own logic. *Nursing Outlook, 50*, 204–212.

Paterson, J., & Zderad, L. (1976). *Humanistic nursing*. New York, NY: Wiley.

Peplau, H. (1952). *Interpersonal relations in nursing*. New York, NY: Putnam.

Peplau, H. (1992). Interpersonal relations: A theoretical framework for application in nursing practice. *Nursing Science Quarterly, 5*, 13–18.

Pickering, A. (1995). *The mangle of practice: Time, agency, and science*. Chicago, IL: University of Chicago.

Pickstone, J. V. (2000). *Ways of knowing: A new history of science, technology and medicine*. Manchester, United Kingdom: Manchester University Press.

Raymo, C. (2006). *Walking zero: Discovering cosmic space and time along the Prime Meridian*. New York, NY: Walker.

Reed, P. G. (1996). Transforming practice knowledge into nursing knowledge—A revisionist analysis of Peplau. *Image: Journal of Nursing Scholarship, 28*(1), 27–31.

Reed, P. G. (2006). The practice turn in nursing epistemology. *Nursing Science Quarterly, 19*(1), 36–38.

Rolfe, G. (1996). *Closing the theory–practice gap: A new paradigm for nursing*. Oxford, United Kingdom: Butterworth-Heinemann.

Rolfe, G. (2000). *Nursing praxis and the reflexive practitioner: Collected papers 1993–1999*. London, England: Nursing Praxis International.

Rouse, J. (2002). *How scientific practices matter*. Chicago, IL: University of Chicago Press.

Roy, C., & Obloy, M. (1978). The practitioner movement—Toward a science of nursing. *American Journal of Nursing, 10,* 1698–1702.

Schatzki, T. R., Cetina, K. K., & von Savigny, E. (Eds.). (2001). *The practice turn in contemporary theory.* New York, NY: Routledge.

Shusterman, R. (1997). *Practicing philosophy: Pragmatism and the philosophical life.* New York, NY: Routledge.

Index